An Inquiry Concerning
GROWTH, DISEASE
AND AGEING

An Inquiry Concerning

GROWTH, DISEASE
AND AGEING

PHILIP R. J. BURCH, M.A., Ph.D.

Deputy Director, Medical Research Council
Environmental Radiation Research Unit

Honorary Reader, Department of
Medical Physics, The University of Leeds

UNIVERSITY OF TORONTO PRESS

OLIVER AND BOYD LTD
Tweeddale Court
14 High Street
Edinburgh 1

First published in Canada and the United States 1969
by University of Toronto Press
SBN 8020 1604 9
© P. R. J. Burch

Printed in Great Britain by
Aberdeen University Press

PREFACE AND ACKNOWLEDGEMENTS

Tycho Brahe's meticulous observations paved the way firstly for Kepler's empirical laws of planetary motion, and then for Newton's all-embracing law of gravitation. Scientific knowledge advances from the particular to the general. In the nineteenth century, Darwin and Mendel hammered out two great generalisations in biology. Currently, biochemists, molecular biologists and biophysicists create new synopses at the molecular level. But in the more classical areas of biology and medicine multitudinous details accumulate. This harvesting of data encourages intensive specialisation, and the existence of over 2,000 medical journals. We seem to be approaching the stage of one consultant, one disease.

Although specialisation generated many of the studies exploited in this book, my main purpose is to emphasise, not their separateness and diversity, but their underlying unity. Following Professor Burwell, I contend that a central homoeostatic system regulates the normal growth of tissues, throughout the body. This same growth-control system breaks down, in highly specific ways, to initiate a vast range of apparently unconnected diseases and conditions of ageing.

General laws of a mathematical character adorn modern physics. With the notable exception of Mendel's laws of inheritance, biology lacks these precise formulations. I argue, however, that unifying laws, akin to those of physics, describe some of the most fundamental features of growth and of pathology. Critical and testable predictions follow from these laws.

My indebtedness to many colleagues and collaborators, but especially to Professor R. G. Burwell, Dr F. T. de Dombal, Mr C. G. Fairpo, Professor D. Jackson, Dr N. R. Rowell, and Dr D. Taverner will be obvious from the text; I deeply appreciate the generous support of Professor F. W. Spiers. Any clarity which the book may possess owes much to my wife Dr Jane E. Burch who carefully vetted, and greatly improved the original manuscript. Dr Janet Moore, Dr J. A. Sharp and

Dr D. Tarin also provided valuable and constructive criticisms. Miss Anne Taylor has given excellent secretarial help, and Mr H. G. Lumby carefully prepared the line drawings.

I am grateful to the following editors and publishers for permission to reproduce the indicated figures: the Editor of the *British Dental Journal* (Figs 3.2 and 3.3); the Editors and publishers, Edinburgh University Press, of *Rheumatic Diseases* (Figs 4.2 and 4.3); the Editor of the *Journal of Bone and Joint Surgery*, British Edition (Fig. 4.4); the Editors and publishers, Taylor and Francis Ltd, of *Radiation and Ageing* (Figs 4.5, 4.7, 4.9, 4.10, 4.19, 4.20, 4.22 and 7.2); the Editor of the *British Journal of Psychiatry* (Figs 4.11, 4.12 and 4.13); and the Editors and publishers, North-Holland Publishing Co., of the *Handbook of Clinical Neurology* (Fig. 7.1).

CONTENTS

1. INTRODUCTION: SCOPE AND DEFINITIONS

'Despite the reluctance of many physicians to extend the concept of autoimmune disease beyond the conditions in which antibody against some body component is clearly demonstrable, there is a growing trend to look for an autoimmune component in a wide range of subacute and chronic conditions.'

Sir Macfarlane Burnet, 1961

We all age. In real life there are no Peter Pans. But even without the aid of cosmetics some of us look young for our years, while others, for no obvious reasons, acquire a venerable mien by the age of 40. Some people resent being heirs to mortal flesh and crave for the elixir of life. Others are able to reconcile themselves with dignity to the inevitability of senescence and death. But the degree of our philosophical detachment is apt to be influenced by the particular diseases and ailments that afflict us, and the severity, extent, and duration of our pains. Suffering may purge the soul, but twentieth-century man finds more consolation in the thought that another thousand million dollars to the National Institutes of Health might rid him of his backache.

Despite the omnipresence of the ageing process (we are lucky if we have not lost a tooth) the scientific study of ageing – that is gerontology – is a fairly new discipline, and it has only recently achieved respectability. In this book I shall not attempt to give a comprehensive review of the evidence and theories relating to ageing because this has already been done by several authors, and notably by Comfort (1964). Instead, I shall describe in some detail, a unitary theory of growth and disease. This relates the physiological phenomena of growth-control and cellular differentiation to many aberrant and pathological phenomena, including the so-called 'autoimmune' diseases and ageing.

My thesis has its roots in Sir Macfarlane Burnet's 'forbidden-clone' theory of disturbed-tolerance autoimmunity. This concept, like so many of the really great ideas, is in essence very simple, and a short excursion into immunology will suffice to explain it.

THE IMMUNOLOGICAL PROBLEM OF 'SELF-RECOGNITION'

Burnet has persistently emphasised that the main challenge confronting immunologists is the problem of self-tolerance or 'self-recognition'. In health, our complex immune system respects our own normal cells and tissues; the antibodies we synthesise do not attack them. On the other hand, if we introduce into our body 'not-self' material such as bacteria or viruses, or if we attempt to graft a piece of skin, say, from another person onto ourself, then our complex immune system quickly recognises the foreignness of these extrinsic substances and it reacts to them in various ways. An extremely versatile mechanism, the nature of which will be explored in the ensuing chapters, somehow distinguishes 'self' from 'not-self'. The outer coat of a bacterium or virus carries molecular structures that are capable of binding antibody; such structures are called antigens. These antigens are identified by the host; the resulting complexes are phagocytised; and the invading micro-organisms are destroyed. Antibodies combining with 'classical' antigens of this kind, are to be found in the immuno-globulin – mainly IgA, IgG and IgM – plasma protein fractions. Our lymphoid system can also recognise the alien nature of the skin graft, which is usually rejected in about two weeks. Small lymphocytes are generally believed to be important to graft rejection, while the contribution of humoral immunoglobulin antibodies to this process is obscure.

This complexity of immune mechanisms presents some awkward terminological problems. The expression *lymphoid system* is usually taken to refer to lymphoid cells in the bone marrow, to organs such as the thymus, spleen, and lymph nodes, to subepithelial lymphoid tissue, lymphatics, and circulating lymphocytes. It includes cells which synthesise and secrete immunoglobulins. As we shall see later, I often need to refer to particular sections of the lymphoid system together with comparable sections of the granulocytic series of cells which, I shall argue, are primarily concerned not with classical immunity, but with the much more fundamental function of growth-control. I shall adopt expressions which emphasise these distinctions.

One important exception to the graft-rejection phenomenon must be mentioned. If you happen to be one of a pair of identical twins, and if a piece of skin from your twin is carefully grafted onto yourself, then in health you will accept this graft. In other words, you tolerate it. This implies that the recognition of foreign tissues depends upon the existence of a *genetic* difference between the donor tissue and the host. Monozygotic (identical) twins have the same genetic make-up – somatic mutations apart – and a tissue from one twin 'looks like' self-tissue to the lymphoid system of the other twin. Accordingly, it is not rejected; it is accepted as 'self' (but see Chapter 9). The molecular configurations, or antigens, on the plasma (outer) membrane of a given kind of cell, have the same structure and specificity in both members of a monozygotic twin pair because they are coded by genes which have their origin in a single cell, that is, the common zygote. Certain of these antigens on the plasma membrane are called *histo-compatibility* (or *histoincompatibility*) antigens.

The genetic basis of the distinction between self and not-self has been amply confirmed in animal experiments, where it is possible to work with highly inbred strains in which individual animals of a given sex are genetically identical, or very nearly so, with all other individuals of that strain. (Significantly, tissues from XY male animals carry some antigens that are never found in female tissues, because they are coded by, and synthesised under the direction of, genes on the Y-chromosome.) Grafting experiments show that the severity of the reaction of the host towards the donor tissue depends upon the nature of the genetic differences between the donor and host animals: genes at some histocompatibility loci are far more important in this respect than others.

Rejection follows, it is widely believed, when the cellular antigens of the graft are incompatible with certain cells of the host's lymphoid system. Our theory predicts that, in certain situations, incompatibility with humoral products of the host's basophil series of cells will also be important to graft injury and/or rejection. (See Chapters 9 and 10.) We shall now consider briefly what might happen if the mechanism of self-recognition should fail.

FAILURE OF SELF-RECOGNITION

The simplest type of failure which can be imagined is a change in the antigenicity of, say, a skin cell. Because the configuration and therefore specificity of cellular antigens is ultimately determined by genes, let us suppose that spontaneous or induced gene changes occur in one of my skin cells so that it becomes identical with many of your skin cells. We have seen that because you are not my identical twin, I shall generally reject a graft of your skin. By analogy therefore, I should 'reject' or destroy any of my own skin cells which, through mutation, have become genetically and phenotypically identical with yours. Fortunately, I can readily dispense with the occasional skin cell, and hence genetic changes leading to the loss of only a small proportion of such cells would be of little or no consequence. The loss would soon be replaced through the mitosis of normal cells, as in wound repair. Nevertheless, other kinds of gene mutations in skin or other cells can be imagined which would lead, not to cellular destruction, but to neoplastic and malignant change. Some references will be made to the problem of cancer, but the subject is too vast and unresolved to be discussed in detail in this book. However, the close connection between leukaemia, Burkitt's lymphoma, and Hodgkin's disease on the one hand, and 'autoimmunity' on the other, will be considered in Chapter 11.

We must now turn to an even more important aspect of failure in self-recognition. In the course of his disquisition on the nature of self-tolerance, Burnet considered the possible consequences of spontaneous or induced gene changes not only in 'target' cells, but also in the stem cells of the lymphoid system. This was probably one of the most momentous steps in the history of medicine. Unless many of us are badly mistaken, it holds the key to the understanding not only of recognised 'autoimmune' disease, but also of many of the phenomena of ageing.

FORBIDDEN-CLONE THEORY OF DISEASE

Burnet argued that gene change in a mesenchymal stem cell might give rise to the growth of a clone of cells, whose *autoantibody* products react with self tissues. (Autoantibodies are antibodies synthesised by one's own cells which attack, or combine specifically with, antigenic determinants of tissues, cells, or molecules, forming a part of oneself.) The mutations in the stem cell destroy the genetic basis of normal self-tolerance. Through the process of repeated cell-division the faulty or mutant stem cell propagates a large number of similar descendant cells, each one of which inherits, and is therefore tainted by, the faults of its progenitor. These clonal cells, or their secreted 'mutant' antibody products, circulate through the body and attack any cells carrying complementary antigenic determinants. Burnet describes this clone of faulty cells synthesising either humoral or cellular autoantibodies, as a *forbidden-clone*. He calls its growth a *conditioned malignancy* (Burnet 1965).

Attacked cells react in a variety of ways to the assault by autoantibodies, and colleagues and I have argued that all the 'classical' autoimmune diseases result from the formation and proliferation of one or more forbidden-clones. We have also proposed that, in certain instances, the outcome is a change which we normally think of as a feature of ageing.

WHAT IS AGEING?

Many attempts have been made to formulate definitions that might command general acceptance, and much space could be devoted to discussing their merits and limitations. By and large I think the space would be wasted. Precise definition is sometimes essential to the development of a science, and in the present context I believe that instead of defining the term 'ageing' we should first describe the conditions we are interested in – say the loss of teeth, the greying of hair, the 'hardening' of arteries, the psychoses of senescence, etc. – with all the clinical and diagnostic precision we can command. Having done that we can then try to discover their causes. If ultimately we find that some general type of mechanism is common to most of these different diseases and ageing conditions, we might then be justified in describing it as an ageing mechanism.

What should we exclude from the umbrella term of 'ageing'? Embryogenesis, foetal development, normal growth, puberty and maturation are unquestionably among the most outstanding of age-dependent phenomena. Normally, each stage of development succeeds the previous one in an invariant sequence, and the entire programme of growth and development is triggered by the fertilisation of a female germ cell by a male one. Given adequate nutrition, freedom from maternal infection (especially rubella–German measles), and other interfering agents such as the drug thalidomide, the course is mapped in the main by the initial complement of genes in the zygote. Development is an age-dependent process *par excellence* but I shall not choose to treat it under the term 'ageing' which connotes degenerative processes and senescence. Unfortunately, the semantic snare cannot be escaped quite as easily as this, because the evidence shows that degenerative processes can start, and in some rare instances they can even terminate life, as early as the foetal stage. However, the kind of degenerative process I shall discuss is associated in its overt form *predominantly*, though not exclusively, with old age; its occurrence during development is not a necessary part of that process; it represents an unfortunate breakdown of the normal mechanism.

CONNECTION BETWEEN GROWTH-CONTROL, 'AUTOIMMUNE' DISEASE AND AGEING

It would be convenient to leave the discussion of scope and definitions at this point but I am hindered by a fundamental consideration. In 1963, my then colleague in Leeds, Dr R. Geoffrey Burwell, proposed that the primary and *intrinsic* function of the lymphoid system is none other than that of the control of growth. Incredulous when Burwell first acquainted me with his ideas, I was eventually persuaded by my own studies, in conjunction with his resourceful advocacy, that his revolutionary notions are basically correct. Furthermore, it transpired that the so-called 'autoimmune' diseases and many forms of ageing, result – at least in our view – from a particular form of breakdown in the mechanism of central growth-control. I am therefore compelled to describe (see Chapters 6 and 11) the essential features of the postulated central growth-control system, although its *normal* functioning belongs to physiology, and not pathology.

Terminological difficulties emerge again. Immunoglobulin *auto*-antibodies – the same type of molecular species as classical immune antibodies – can often be detected in patients with certain diseases, and it has been widely assumed that such autoantibodies are the primary causal agents. Because these autoantibodies are synthesised by lymphoid and plasma cells of the classical immune system, the associated disorders have been, and are still generally called, *autoimmune* diseases. We are confident, however, that immunoglobulin autoantibodies are not the primary cause of such diseases. Normal immuno-globulins do not regulate growth (see next chapter). We would prefer to substitute the term *autoaggressive* for *autoimmune*, and in the main I shall use this new terminology.

Where degenerative change is concerned I shall confine the discussion to conditions that are manifested at the macroscopic level. Innumerable changes presumably occur at the micro-scopic and sub-microscopic levels which have no substantial influence on the general economy of the body. These will not detain us. On the other hand, those sub-microscopic events that lead to macroscopic effects will occupy much of our attention.

In short, I shall present a unified theory of many physio-logical and pathological phenomena that, hitherto, have not been clearly connected. I shall attempt to link central growth control, cellular differentiation, immune mechanisms, and some forms of genetic polymorphism to those many disease and ageing conditions that contribute to the ill-health, unhappiness, and impoverishment of mankind.

2. ORIGINS OF THE UNIFIED THEORY

'Possibly in the last resort the control of cell growth has an immunological basis.'

H. N. Green, 1959

Green published the first immunological theory of cancer in 1954. He pioneered the view that cancer represents a breakdown in cell recognition.

IMMUNOLOGICAL ASPECTS OF CANCER

Normal cells, according to Green, are characterised by *'identity proteins'*, and their loss constitutes *in itself* the neoplastic change: the gradations and progression of neoplasia correspond to the extent of their loss. Green (1954) believed that chemical carcinogens produce a highly specific antigenic change in the 'identity proteins', and the immune response to this alteration represents the primary stage in chemical carcinogenesis.

This theory, together with Burnet's (1957, 1959, 1961) insistence on the need to explain the antigenic distinction between 'self' and 'not-self', strongly influenced my own thinking, and I incorporated these basic recognition concepts in a general theory of cancer formation (Burch 1963a,b). Malignant cells have of course escaped from normal growth-control, but it is a widely recognised principle that insight into physiological mechanisms can often be gained by studying the details of their breakdown. I proposed that the pre-malignant cell harbours multiple mutant genes which are mainly acquired, although some of them are often inherited. Certain of these mutant genes code for the synthesis of altered or 'not-self' proteins. These 'mutant' proteins form a part of the plasma membrane of the cells (as well as a part of a cytoplasmic membrane network called the endoplasmic reticulum) and they render the cell autoantigenic to the host's immunological recognition apparatus.

Following Green (1954, 1958), I argued that the pre-malignant autoantigenic cell is generally converted to the malignant state through one or more specific interactions with complementary humoral or cellular antibodies. This type of disturbed-antigen autoimmune interaction would normally be expected to result in the destruction of the mutant cell; but the premalignant cell is mutant in a particularly vicious way, and instead of being destroyed, it gains its freedom. Metabolic pathways are switched from the resting (non-dividing) phase, and they eventually become 'locked' into the mitotic phase; the character of the plasma membrane is to all intents and purposes irreversibly changed and fully malignant growth proceeds.

Viewed in this way, cancer is a special form of *disturbed-antigen*, as opposed to *disturbed-tolerance* autoimmune disease. The changes that initiate the disease process occur in cells of tissue that becomes the target of 'immune' attack, but instead of being killed by complementary antibody, the premalignant cell escapes into runaway growth.

THE LYMPHOID SYSTEM AND THE CONTROL OF NORMAL GROWTH

This theory of the genesis of cancer attracted the attention of my colleague Burwell. His main concern however was not with malignancy but with normal growth. He had been studying changes in regional lymph nodes draining bone grafts (Burwell 1962, 1964), and he observed, among other things, that the reaction pattern following an allograft was not the same as that which followed a xenograft. (An allograft or homograft is a graft of tissue from an animal of the same species, but of a different genotype or strain from the host; a xenograft is a graft from an animal of a different species.) Many other investigators had made similar observations but Burwell proceeded to a brilliant induction. He first deduced that humoral factors flowed from the foreign tissue to the regional lymph node draining the graft, while graft-rejection, long recognised as an immunological phenomenon (Medawar 1946) showed that antibodies of some kind, complementary to the graft, travelled in the reverse direction. Burwell then reasoned that if such afferent and efferent pathways exist under these artificial experimental conditions, they must surely be present under natural, physiological conditions, as well. What then is their physiological function?

According to Burwell (1963), *the intrinsic function of the lymphoid system is none other than that of growth-control.* In addition to being a policeman, apprehending the breaking-and-entering bacterium or virus, or objecting to the presence of the alien transplanted kidney, a part of the ubiquitous lymphoid system assumes the role of supreme commander, directing our growth, and governing our size. Ultimately it breaks down and destroys us. In my opinion, this remarkable proposal – or more strictly, certain general principles which follow from it – could prove to be one of the great stepping stones to an understanding of the biology of multi-tissue organisms. (I shall argue later that the lymphoid system is not the only one involved in central growth-control in mammals: basophilic granulocytes appear also to be implicated. In any case, invertebrates have no lymphoid tissue.)

Burwell expounded his revolutionary ideas shortly after the publication of my cancer theory, and he told me that the interaction of 'antibody' with target cells is responsible, not only for initiating mitosis in premalignant cells – as I had just argued – but also for promoting mitosis in *normal* cells. I must confess that I was initially outraged by this heretical doctrine, and I carefully explained that it is the *foreignness* – the autoantigenic property – of the premalignant cell that attracts the attention of antibodies. A complementary antibody recognises and fastens itself onto the autoantigenic membrane of the premalignant cell. The special characteristic of the normal non-mutant cell is that it is non-antigenic; a state of tolerance and *non-interaction* exists between it and the normal products of the lymphoid system – or so I thought at that time when I was firmly wedded to the clonal selection theory of acquired immunity (Burnet 1957, 1959). In Burnet's view, which I still share, the central challenge of immunology is the biological basis of self-tolerance: how does the lymphoid system distinguish between the innumerable constituents of self – which it normally tolerates – and the even more numerous examples of not-self, with which it reacts in various and complex ways?

SELF-RECOGNITION

Burnet's clonal selection theory provided an ingenious solution to this classical problem which engrossed Ehrlich and many of his successors. During embryogenesis, according to Burnet, mutations occur at a high frequency in the antibody-coding genes of presumptive stem cells in the mesenchymal system. The polypeptide chain products of these hypermutable genes make up a wide range of antibody specificities. If by chance an antibody should emerge that reacts with exposed antigens of self tissues, then a homoeostatic monitor is supposed to identify and to eliminate cells synthesising self-reacting *auto*antibodies. At the end of this embryonic phase, our antibodies should therefore be able to recognise many foreign antigens, while the relation of our antibody-producing cells, and their products, to our normal tissues should be one of indifference. In Burnet's scheme, self-recognition is therefore negative in character. Our antibodies simply *fail* to interact with our own tissues.

In utter contrast, Burwell was postulating that certain products of the lymphoid system react specifically with cells of self-tissues to stimulate them to mitosis. By regulating cell division, a part of the lymphoid system controls and co-ordinates growth. In Burwell's scheme, self-recognition is therefore positive in nature.

At that early stage neither Burwell nor I had conceived of a recognition mechanism based on a non-complementary molecular interaction, and I was not then prepared to abandon Burnet's clonal selection idea, which, with its corollary of mutant or forbidden-clones, accounted both for (negative) self-recognition in health, and autoimmune clashes in disease. Indeed, I protested that Burwell's scheme left no room for autoimmunity. If *normal* lymphoid cells or their humoral products were complementary to normal tissue cells, then how could autoimmune relations – also based on molecular complementarity – ever develop? The deadlock between us was almost complete. I had no satisfactory theory of normal growth-control, and Burwell gave no plausible account of the distinction between a normal mitogenic interaction, and a pathogenic autoimmune attack.

But events were moving swiftly. It so happened that I was

then studying evidence relating to the so-called 'autoimmune' diseases, and I had already encountered a situation that is exceptional in science. Some important statistical properties of such diseases were proving to be far *simpler* than I had anticipated.

RELEVANCE OF STATISTICS OF AUTOAGGRESSIVE DISEASES TO THEORIES OF GROWTH-CONTROL

It soon emerged that the age-distributions of the onset or prevalence of 'autoimmune' diseases, together with various ageing conditions and diseases of unknown cause, agree with the view that they are initiated by a small number of random events. I shall argue later (Chapter 7) that these events are a rather special form of somatic mutation. This stochastic interpretation of the initiating process conformed perfectly with Burnet's (1959) forbidden-clone theory of auto-immunity which I was engaged in testing. One, or several random and rare gene mutations in a mesenchymal stem cell, should be all that is needed to initiate the growth of a forbidden-clone of cells. The descendant mutant cells in the clone, or their humoral products, attack and damage target cells carrying complementary antigenic determinants. An enormous number of skin cells for example, in anatomically dispersed sites, can be simultaneously affected in an 'autoimmune' disease such as chronic discoid lupus erythematosus, and it is difficult to argue (without a good deal of speciousness) that three or four mutations, in one or a few *skin* cells, could be responsible for such widespread and multiple lesions. But we can readily understand how a few random events could trigger a central change, and through *clonal proliferation* could give rise to simultaneous auto-immune attacks on, say, several joints, or arteries, or teeth, or patches of skin.

Although it was interesting and even important to discover that 'autoimmune' diseases are probably initiated by only a few random events, it was far from puzzling because it verified Burnet's prediction. The puzzle resided in the quantitative properties of these events. I had expected to find: (a) in general, the average rate of a specific somatic mutation, estimated on a per unit time basis, would increase during postnatal growth, because I believed the number of stem cells at mutational risk would also increase with the growth of the organism; (b) rates would be rather higher in males than in females, because males, on the average, are larger than females; and (c) the average somatic mutation-rates observed for a general population would represent the mean value for many heterogeneous groups, some with high rates, and others with intermediate or low rates. To my great surprise the more data I examined, the more they refused to conform to any of these common-sense expectations; instead, they fitted a much simpler model which is described in Chapters 3 to 7. In particular the mutation rates, estimated in terms of mutant events per person, per *unit time*, remain remarkably constant throughout growth, suggesting that the number of cells at mutational risk also remains constant throughout postnatal life.

HOMOEOSTATIC CONTROL: BASIC REQUIREMENTS

The wholly unexpected conclusions drawn from age-distribution analysis slowly generated a most uncomfortable suspicion: my verbal sparring partner might be right after all. Suppose certain sections of the mesenchymal system really do regulate the growth and size of tissues. Then some form of negative-feedback relation must be involved, and the central control must be able to 'measure' the size of the growing target tissue. It follows that the central control must contain some kind of fixed 'yard-stick' (a comparator) and it must be able to 'decide' whether the tissue has grown enough.

A *negative* feedback system requires not only a comparator but also *phase-reversal*. That is to say if the target organ is too big, the excess rate of flow of afferent signals from it (indicating its size) must serve to inhibit the release of mitogenic effectors from the central control organ. This phenomenon of inhibition is often found in biochemistry and other regions of biology, and it is easy to understand how afferent signals could either inhibit the maturation of a cell to a mitogenic effector, or inhibit the secretion from a cell of mitogenic macromolecules. We call the mitogenic effectors from the central control organ: *mitotic control proteins* (MCPs). These can be *cellular*, forming probably an integral part of the plasma membrane of one class of small lymphocyte. When target tissues lie behind blood-tissue barriers, the MCPs must be *humoral* rather than cellular: they appear generally to migrate on immunoelectrophoresis with

NEGATIVE FEEDBACK CONTROL OF THE GROWTH OF A TARGET TISSUE BY A CENTRAL CONTROL SYSTEM

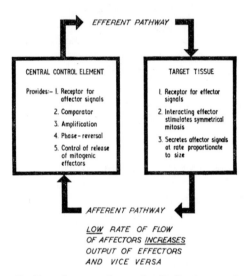

Fig. 2.1 Outline of proposed negative-feedback control of symmetrical mitosis, growth, and the maintenance of the size of target tissues during maturity. Each distinctive target tissue has its own lymphocytic or granulocytic control element. Probably, a series of feedback loops connects control stem cells in the bone marrow, via the thymus, and regional lymph nodes, to the target tissue (see Fig. 11.8).

the α_2-macroglobulin serum protein fraction (Burch 1968a). I have proposed that basophilic granulocytes and mast cells are associated with their production, although this remains to be confirmed experimentally (Burch 1968a). Afferent signals, secreted from target cells, are called *tissue coding factors* (TCFs); they are probably lipoproteins.

If the control system is to be accurate, as it undoubtedly is, there must be a large measure of 'amplification' in the central control. Biology can provide this further property very readily through the processes of repeated cell division, and/or regulated protein synthesis.

In the present context, the important requirement is that of the stable *comparator*, against which the size of the target tissue can be measured. It slowly dawned on me that this necessary feature of control circuits provided an elegant explanation for the unexpected though welcome simplicity of the 'autoimmune' statistics. If 'autoimmune' diseases arise from mutations in growth-control stem cells to produce 'mutant' MCPs, and if the number of growth-control stem cells remains constant during postnatal growth, then such groups of cells can be exploited – however indirectly – to serve as the biological comparator for assessing the extent of growth. They could represent the final court of appeal where issues of normal growth and size are concerned. (See Fig. 2.1.)

Although we can now begin to see how the simple statistics of 'autoimmune' diseases can be explained by Burwell's concept of growth-control, an even more formidable problem remains. How does the growth-control effector (MCP) recognise its target tissue, and how does the affector (TCF) identify the correct control element?

TISSUE RECOGNITION IN GROWTH-CONTROL

We know that each organ has a characteristic growth-pattern, and that this can differ strikingly from organ to organ (see Thompson 1952). To cite extreme examples: whereas the full complement of neurons (and of oocytes in females) is present at birth, most organs continue to increase in size until about 20 years of age. Furthermore, when we remove two-thirds of the liver from an experimental animal, it is the remaining liver tissue which regenerates and not the heart, the kidneys, or the skeleton, etc. Evidence of this kind indicates that the growth of each distinctive tissue is *separately controlled*, but that the development and growth of the whole organism is beautifully *co-ordinated*. This mixture of *independence* and of *interrelatedness* between the individual control elements is at first sight almost contradictory. However, the apparent contradiction is easily resolved if the size of each distinctive target tissue throughout the body is regulated by its own mesenchymal element, containing a fixed number of stem cells. Each control element can then act independently of all the others – because it has a biochemical and 'immunological' separateness – but after a certain stage of embryonic development, the constant number of stem cells in each element necessarily bears a fixed numerical relation to the constant number of stem cells in every other growth-control compartment.

At this early stage of the story I must make an interpolation concerning the fundamental distinction (see Osgood 1957, 1964) between two types of cell division: symmetrical and asymmetrical. Consider the epidermis. When the horny layer is removed, as is continually happening in the course of normal wear and tear, it has to be replaced by the outward migration of underlying cells. These in turn have to be replaced by new cells arising from the mitosis of cells in the basal layer. Here we have an example of asymmetrical cell division where one cell in the basal layer divides to give: (a) one basal layer cell; and (b) another cell migrating outwards. In this form of cell division the number of cells in the basal layer is therefore conserved. The detailed nature of the homoeostatic controls that regulate, say, the thickness of the epidermis or the level of circulating red blood cells – both of which involve asymmetrical mitosis – is unknown. Possibly, the tissue-specific '*chalones*' investigated by Bullough (see Bullough (1965) for a review) are implicated in the regulation of asymmetrical cell division, but I shall make no attempt to discuss this phenomenon here. Instead, I shall turn to symmetrical mitosis.

During normal growth, the total area of the skin increases greatly, and hence the total number of cells in the basal layer of the epidermis must also increase greatly because the size of the individual cells remains more-or-less unaltered. Consequently, a basal layer cell must sometimes divide during growth to give two daughter basal layer cells. This is symmetrical division. We postulate that it is regulated by the central mesenchymal growth-control mechanism, utilising lymphoid and granulocytic elements, and in later chapters I shall discuss certain features of it in some detail.

The sheer complexity of the problem of growth-control is the first thing that strikes us, for we soon realise with Weiss

(1962), that the number of distinctive tissues, and therefore of individual growth-control elements in a complex organism such as man, must be astronomical. Picture the enormously elaborate architecture of the kidneys, the skeleton, and the brain; inspect your own genetically-determined fingerprints. Every regular morphological subtlety has to be controlled in a very precise way, and ultimately, it has to be related to gene action. A vivid illustration of tissue specificity is provided by the regeneration in fish of the experimentally-severed optic nerve (see Gaze's 1967 review). After the nerve has been cut, regenerative growth of the fibres occurs, and usually each central fibre rejoins with the correct retinal element, so that normal vision is restored. Similarly, in the healing of complex wounds, which will involve some measure of symmetrical mitosis, it is found that each distinctive tissue re-unites with its own kind; when fusion has occurred further expansion is arrested (see Weiss 1947 and Chapter 6).

I shall later attempt to define in more detail what I mean by 'distinctive tissues' but on any reckoning their number must be vast. It could well be around 10^8 – give or take an order of magnitude or two (see Chapter 10). Even if the number is as small as 10^6 – which, in view of the specificity of fibres in the optic nerve of fish seems excessively improbable – we are still confronted with a formidable recognition problem. How does the mitogenic effector (MCP) stimulating symmetrical mitosis pick out its appropriate target cell? To compound the difficulty, we see that this is a two-way problem. The TCF affectors from the target tissue – indicating its size – also have to locate their correct growth-control element.

Having viewed this two-way recognition problem with some apprehension, it was a great relief to find that the 'autoimmune' evidence contained a solution to this enigma as well. Arguments deriving from the 'autoimmune' evidence concerning the nature of self-recognition in growth-control, together with others deriving from independent considerations, are deployed in Chapter 6. Briefly, in place of the complementarity relation of the classical antigen-antibody reaction, we deduce that mutual recognition in the central growth-control system relies upon *identity* relations between interacting macromolecules. London-van der Waal's *self-recognition* forces (see Jehle 1963), would appear to provide the physico-chemical basis of mutual recognition in biological growth-control (Burch and Burwell 1965).

With the vexing recognition problem out of the way, the final obstacle to accepting the essence of Burwell's thesis was now removed. Although many details remained to be elucidated – and they still do – I capitulated before the end of 1963.

THE NEED FOR REASSESSMENT

A complete re-orientation of outlook was now called for. Immunoglobulins, the molecular species that are primarily involved in the classical immune response to invading micro-organisms, cannot be the MCPs responsible for growth-control. The Bruton (sex-linked) form of congenital hypo-gammaglobulinaemia (a condition in which circulating immunoglobulins are grossly deficient or absent) is associated with almost normal growth – apart from the absence of plasma cells. Neither can immunoglobulins provide the 'mutant' MCPs that are the primary cause of 'autoimmune' disease, because such conditions occur very commonly both in congenital and acquired hypogammaglobulinaemia (Good *et al.* 1962; Green and Sperber 1962). What then is the connection between classical immunity, immediate and delayed hyper-sensitivity, host-versus-graft and graft-versus-host reactions, and central growth-control? What is the relation between immunoglobulin autoantibodies and 'autoimmune' disease?

I contend that an intrinsic function of immunoglobulins is that of *defence* against proliferating forbidden-clones (Burch 1963c and Chapters 4, 9 and 10). Immediate hypersensitivity is interpreted as an inappropriate response of the humoral growth-control system, and delayed hypersensitivity as an inappropriate response of the cellular growth-control mechanism to specific antigenic challenges (Burch and Burwell 1967, and Chapter 9).

We argue that TCFs, besides being secreted in humoral form to act as affectors in growth-control, also form an integral part of the plasma membrane of target cells: they include histocompatibility antigens (Burch and Burwell 1965). Graft-versus-host and host-versus-graft reactions occur when there is complementarity between MCPs on the one side, and histo-*in*compatible TCFs on the other (Burch and Burwell 1965, 1967 and Chapters 9 and 10).

When we begin our search for a biological system capable of recognising the minutiae of molecular configuration, we first turn to the classical immune system, because the extreme specificity of the affinity between antigen and antibody is its hallmark. As early as 1947, Tyler published a paper 'An auto-antibody concept of cell structure, growth and differentiation'. The opening sentence of this paper provides an apt summary: 'The concept that I wish to present here is that the various molecular substances that form the basis of cell structure bear the same sort of relationship to one another as do antigen and antibody.' Paul Weiss has often used the antigen-antibody analogy to explain specific interactions between cells (see, for example, Weiss 1947, 1950, 1955, 1962) and his *template-antitemplate* mechanism of growth-control (Weiss and Kavanau 1957) is formally analogous to the antigen-antibody rela-tion. The quotation at the head of this chapter; 'Possibly in the last resort the control of cell growth has an immuno-logical basis' is taken from Green's contribution to a Ciba Symposium discussion in 1959. In 1962 Burnet wrote: 'Very recently there have been a number of indications that immuno-logical recognition may be derived from an aspect of the pro-cesses by which multicellular animals succeed in maintaining a characteristic morphological and functional unity. In its most general formulation this capacity must involve an interchange of "information" between cells. A cell seems to be able to "recognise" whether another cell is in contact with it or not and in some instances whether the adjacent cell is of its own type or another' (Burnet 1962).

Many authors have therefore alerted us to the overwhelming importance of specific recognition mechanisms in growth-control and morphology.

3. THEORIES OF AGEING IN RELATION TO AGE-PATTERNS OF DISEASE

'So the living and the dead, things animate and inanimate, we dwellers in the world and this world wherein we dwell . . . are bound alike by physical and mathematical law.'

D'Arcy Wentworth Thompson

Two highly contrasted approaches to the problem of ageing have enjoyed considerable popularity. At one extreme ageing is said to be a programmed phenomenon, timed by an internal device formally resembling a clock. We can regard the sequential loss of oocytes from the ovary as an example of this kind of mechanism. (However, for reasons explained in detail elsewhere (Burch and Rowell 1963; Burch and Gunz 1967), the onset of the menopause is unlikely to be timed by a non-random sequential, or clock-like mechanism.) The programmed view of ageing is an extension of the preformationist concept of development and growth, and it regards senescence as that preordained stage which follows the attainment of maturity.

At the opposite extreme, natural ageing is regarded as a purely stochastic phenomenon resulting from the accumulation of random 'errors'. This view is usually linked with the concept of somatic mutation, entailing spontaneous or induced gene-change, or chromosomal-defect, in somatic cells. One version of the somatic mutation theory holds that the accumulation of gene changes or chromosomal aberrations in *fixed post-mitotic cells* is responsible for ageing. A good example of fixed post-mitotic cells is provided by neurons (nerve cells) which in man show no normal mitotic activity after birth. Proponents of this theory of ageing believe that errors accumulated in this type of cell lead to malfunctioning and gradual degenerative change. Even when the altered cell is completely lost, it cannot be replaced by the mitosis of unaltered cells of a similar differentiation, because by definition they are also fixed post-mitotic cells.

The main postulates of this theory – the occurrence of gene and chromosomal mutation in fixed post-mitotic cells, followed by cellular malfunctioning and degeneration at the *microscopic level* – are well supported experimentally (Curtis 1966) and they would seem to be incontestable. However, it by no means follows that the deterioration of individual chromosomes and cells arising in this way is responsible for the overt *macroscopic* changes of senescence. The situation resembles the loss of the occasional skin cell, cited in Chapter 1. Provided the proportion of cells lost is small, and provided losses are randomly distributed, no significant ill-effects will accrue. By and large, a measure of cellular redundancy in the typical mammal provides a form of buffering, or insurance, against the occasional loss of individual cells. We concede however that dermal cells, and the basal cells of the epidermis, are not fixed post-mitotic cells, and hence their loss – when inflicted by wounds – can generally be made good through mitosis of healthy cells. Indeed, if ageing were confined to changes in fixed post-mitotic cells, it would be difficult to understand how the skin could age at all – but it undoubtedly does.

In a purely formal sense, the disturbed-tolerance 'auto-immune' (autoaggressive) theory of ageing lies between the two extreme view-points described above: it combines stochastic with sequential features (Burch and Jackson 1966b). Briefly, the emergence of an autoaggressive condition in a genetically-predisposed person can be divided into two broad phases: *initiation*, which is a purely stochastic phenomenon normally involving spontaneous somatic mutations; and *progression*, which is in part a sequential phenomenon, although accidental environmental factors may accelerate this phase, and therapeutic measures may retard it.

PREDICTED AGE-DISTRIBUTIONS

These three theories make different predictions concerning the age-distributions of ageing conditions. Consequently, age-patterns provide a critical test of the validity of theories of disease and ageing.

If ageing is a programmed or sequential phenomenon like normal growth, we must assume that its timing will be largely governed by a genetic mechanism. In that case, if we take two individuals with initially identical complements of genes – that is to say monozygotic twins – and if these are brought up in similar environments, we would expect to find that the timing of the onset of any given ageing condition would be almost simultaneous in the co-twins. *Developmental* phenomena such as menstruation, agree strikingly with these expectations. For monozygotic twins, the mean difference in the age at menarche (onset of menstruation) is only 2 to 3 months, whereas for dizygotic twins it is 10 months, and for unrelated women, it is about 19 months (see Burch and Rowell 1963). Hence, under ordinary environmental conditions, the timing of this developmental phenomenon is dominated by genetic factors.

So far as I am aware no fully rigorous studies of this kind have been carried out in connection with ageing and degenerative diseases, although the onset of these conditions often fails to coincide in monozygotic twins.

Investigations of cancer – one important facet of ageing – have shown a typical concordance for monozygotic twins of about 0·1, and a still lower value for dizygotic twins (see Burch 1963a). That is to say, in a group of monozygotic twin pairs where one twin has cancer, the chance that the other twin will also be found to have cancer is about one in ten. The detailed interpretation of such evidence requires a careful study of the sex and age of affected and unaffected twin-pairs, by cancer type. For our present purposes, however, factors determining cancer induction clearly differ from those which time the onset of menstruation and other stages of growth and development.

The available evidence is at variance with the notion that the onset of most ageing and 'autoimmune' conditions in man is determined by a genetically-programmed, or clock-like mechanism.

It is difficult to make accurate quantitative predictions concerning the age-dependence of conditions that might arise from the loss or deterioration of fixed post-mitotic cells. Suppose, however, an ageing phenomenon manifests itself at some arbitrary level of diagnosis when the proportion, f, of deteriorated fixed post-mitotic cells in a given organ, exceeds some threshold level. A degenerative condition might become detectable when, say, more than one-tenth of cells is affected, that is, when $f > 0.1$. Suppose the organ or tissue is a very small one and contains only 10^5 cells. Then the loss or dysfunction of at least 10^4 cells is required to reveal the ageing condition.

If only one random event is needed to impair one cell, then provided the average rate of each event, and the threshold the onset would be almost simultaneous (within a year or so) level of detection, are similar from person to person, in all people. In other words, the distribution of the age of onset of this hypothetical condition would be very narrow indeed. (It would be still narrower for larger organs.) If the mean age at onset was t, then the standard deviation of the distribution would be $\pm t/(10^4)^{\frac{1}{2}}$ which is, $\pm 0.01t$.

I doubt, however, whether any practical diagnostic criterion could distinguish clearly between $f = 0.1$ and, say, $f = 0.103$ or $f = 0.097$. Consequently, practical forms of diagnosis would be expected to yield an age-distribution normal in character, but with a standard deviation greater than $\pm 0.01t$.

Unfortunately for this theory, the age-onset curves for ageing conditions seldom, and perhaps never show a normal distribution. (The menopausal-age comes near to such a distribution (Burch and Gunz 1967) but the exact age-at-onset is difficult to determine, and Way (1954) found strong indications that it is affected by genetic factors. In other words, the general population of women is not homogeneous with respect to the 'timing' of the menopause; it consists of multiple sub-populations, each with its own characteristic age-pattern.) The theory that ageing results from the loss of fixed post-mitotic cells could, however, be rescued by a protracted series of *ad hoc* manoeuvres. We could argue that the average rate of the random events inactivating cells differs from person to person, and/or that the value of f differs. Arbitrary adjustments of these parameters could then be made to fit any observed age-distribution. When a theory is driven to such expedients it is usually ready for retirement. We prefer models that predict the observed age-distribution from a small number of simple and biologically-plausible premises.

Our autoaggressive approach to ageing and disease is described in detail in the next two chapters. The sex- and age-patterns of many diseases and ageing conditions show impressive agreement with theory. Briefly, I show that auto-aggressive ('autoimmune') conditions are initiated by a *small number* of random events. In Chapter 7 I argue that these spontaneous gene changes are a special form of mutation in somatic cells.

I shall now discuss the concept of randomness first in the context of physics (radioactivity), and then in relation to a simple disease process.

RANDOM EVENTS AND RADIOACTIVITY

Radioactive decay provides a good analogy with the postulated gene changes initiating autoaggressive disease. A given nucleus of radium is just as likely to decay by the emission of an α-particle today, as it is tomorrow, or during any other period of 24 hours. The *probability* that it will decay during any specific interval of time is well-defined. Under all ordinary conditions on this planet it is determined solely by the intrinsic structure and instability of the nucleus. Although we cannot predict the actual instant at which any particular nucleus will decay, we can describe accurately the statistics of the decay of a very large number of radium nuclei. If we start off with 1 g of radium today, we know it will take 1600 years for this to decay to 0·5 g radium, another 1600 years to decay to 0·25 g, another 1600 years to decay to 0·125 g, and so on. That is to say, the *half-life* of radium is 1600 years.

If we have a very large number, N, of radioactive nuclei at time t, then the rate of their decay, $-dN/dt$, depends simply on N and the intrinsic instability of each nucleus. In mathematical terms we have:

$$dN/dt = -cN \qquad [3.1]$$

where c is the decay constant of the radioactive nucleus, which is related to the half-life, $T_{\frac{1}{2}}$ as follows:

$$T_{\frac{1}{2}} = \frac{1}{c}\ln 2 \qquad [3.2]$$

Integrating equation [3.1], and expressing the number of undecayed nuclei present at time $t = 0$ as N_0, we have:

$$N = N_0 \exp(-ct) \qquad [3.3]$$

That is to say, the decay of our source of radium with time follows a negative exponential law. Taking natural logarithms of both sides of equation [3.3] we have:

$$\ln \mathcal{N} = \ln \mathcal{N}_0 - ct \qquad [3.4]$$

Combining equations [3.1] and [3.3], or simply by differentiating [3.3], we have:

$$dN/dt = -c\,\mathcal{N}_0 \exp\,(-ct) \qquad [3.5]$$

and hence the rate of disintegration, that is, the intensity of our radioactive source, dN/dt, also falls off with time according to a negative exponential law.

Hence, if we plot the measured intensity of our radioactive source on a logarithmic scale, against time on a linear scale, we obtain a straight line of slope $-c$. This form of graphical presentation is illustrated in Fig. 3.1, although the example is

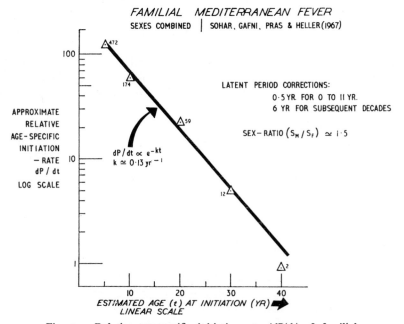

Fig. 3.1   Relative age-specific initiation-rate (dP/dt) of familial Mediterranean fever (on log scale), as a function of the estimated mean age (t) at initiation (on linear scale). From Sohar et al. 1967. For clarity in this and other figures, data are plotted as points instead of histograms; the number of patients in an age-group is indicated alongside a point. The equation of the straight line is $dP/dt \propto \exp\,(-kt)$, where the constant k is 0·13 yr^{-1}.

taken not from physics but from the age-dependence of a disease in man.

The number of atomic nuclei disintegrating between $t = 0$ and $t = t$ is $N_0 - N$, which, from equation [3.3] is:

$$N_0 - N = N_0 \left[1 - \exp \left(-ct \right) \right] \qquad [3.6]$$

Hence the proportion of the original number N_0 of nuclei decaying between $t = 0$ and $t = t$ is:

$$(N_0 - N)/N_0 = 1 - \exp \left(-ct \right) \qquad [3.7]$$

When ct is appreciably less than unity (say 0·1 or below) equation [3.7] approximates very closely to:

$$(N_0 - N)/N_0 = ct \qquad [3.8]$$

That is, at low ct, the proportion of nuclei decaying over a period t, is simply proportional to t. If $(N_0 - N)/N_0$ is plotted on a linear scale, against t on a linear scale, the initial slope of the curve is therefore c, but when ct is much larger than unity, $(N_0 - N)/N_0$ becomes almost unity (nearly all atoms have decayed) and the slope of the curve is almost zero. If $(N_0 - N)/N_0$ is plotted on a logarithmic scale, against t on a similar logarithmic scale, the initial slope of the curve is unity – because $(N_0 - N)/N_0$ increases initially with the *first power* of t – and again, the final slope at high ct is zero. A log–log graph of equation [3.7] is illustrated in Fig. 3.2.

We now turn from physics, and transitions in the nucleus of an atom, to biology, and gene transitions in the nucleus of a cell.

EPIDEMIOLOGY. DEFINITIONS

The *prevalence* of a disorder defines the proportion of people in a population, actually showing present or past evidence of the disorder, at some given moment in time. Frequently, the chance that a person will have a given disease depends on age. To define prevalence in more detail, we need to know the proportion of people, in a given age-range, showing the disease at some given time. This age-specific proportion is defined as *age-specific prevalence*, or more shortly, *age-prevalence*. Convenient age-ranges are: 1 year, 5 years (0 to 4, 5 to 9, 10 to 14, etc.) or 10 years (0 to 9, 10 to 19, 20 to 29, etc.). The choice between them will depend upon factors such as the number of available cases, and the rate of change of prevalence with age, but given large numbers, the narrower the age range, the better. Quite often, sex-differences in age-distributions are found, and then we need to know the proportion of men in given age-ranges, and separately, the proportion of women that are affected. This is *sex-specific and age-specific prevalence*, or more shortly *sex and age prevalence*. Population surveys are used to determine sex and age prevalence.

Many disorders are much too rare to be investigated conveniently through population studies, and in some acute diseases death occurs soon after onset. In such circumstances we have to resort to other evidence for sex and age distributions such as: consecutive patients in a consultant's clinical series, hospital admission statistics for certifiable diseases, and mortality statistics. Provided there is no significant sex or age bias in the selection of data, these sources can provide most valuable evidence for *sex-specific and age-specific onset-rates*, or comparable *mortality-rates*. Suppose that in the years 1958 and 1959, an average of 100 000 men aged 30 to 34 years were alive in a defined population, and suppose that fifty new male cases of disease A arose in this group during the years 1958 and 1959. Then the average age-specific onset-rate of disease A for males aged 30 to 34 years, during the two-year period 1958 and 1959, was: $50/(100\ 000 \times 2)$, or 250 per million, per year. When the absolute size of a population is unknown, and this is common in many clinical series, *relative* sex-specific and age-specific onset-rates can be calculated provided we know the relative sex and age structure of the population from which the patients are drawn.

Most diseases have been progressing for some time before symptoms or signs are detected. In general, an interval called the *latent period* will intervene between the *initiation* of a disease process, and its symptomatic or clinical onset. We can therefore define sex-specific and age-specific *initiation*-rates, and the sex-specific and age-prevalence of *initiated* disease, in the way we define the onset-rates, and prevalence of overt disease.

RANDOM EVENTS AND DISEASE IN MAN

I find that the age-distribution of certain diseases follows the same empirical law as the decay of a radioactive source (Burch 1967d). Thus, the relative age-specific initiation rate (dP/dt) of familial Mediterranean fever, as a function of age, t, can be represented (Fig. 3.1) by the equation:

$$dP/dt = A \exp(-kt) \qquad [3.9]$$

where A is a constant, and the value of the constant k is 0.13 yr^{-1}. Equation [3.9] is exactly equivalent in form to equation [3.5], which describes the rate of disintegration of atomic nuclei in a radioactive source as a function of time.

When a correction is made for latent period, the age-specific mortality (P_t) of first permanent molars (the proportion of lost teeth in a given age-group) is described (Fig. 3.2) by the equation:

$$P_t = 1 - \exp(-kt) \qquad [3.10]$$

The value of the constant k is 0.054 yr^{-1}.

Equation [3.10] is exactly equivalent in form to equation [3.7], which describes the proportion of nuclei which have disintegrated between $t = 0$ and $t = t$.

It is intriguing to find that the age-distributions of these two disorders follow the same empirical law as radioactive decay, but does it mean they are initiated by events that are random in character? Is the agreement with simple stochastic laws a mere coincidence? I pursue these questions in detail in the next three chapters and in Chapter 11. I argue that many diseases are initiated by random events; that the initiating events are a special form of spontaneous somatic gene mutation; and that this kind of interpretation is the best that is available to us. Meanwhile, let us consider whether a biological model based on Burnet's (1959) forbidden-clone theory of autoimmunity, can account for the simple age-distributions of the form [3.9] and [3.10] in Figs 3.1 and 3.2.

Suppose every person in the population has a specific set of cells, the number (L) of which is constant, from around birth to the end of the lifespan; suppose each cell in this set contains a gene which, on mutation, will initiate a particular disease process; and suppose the average rate of mutation of this gene is m, per cell at risk, per year. When one of the L cells

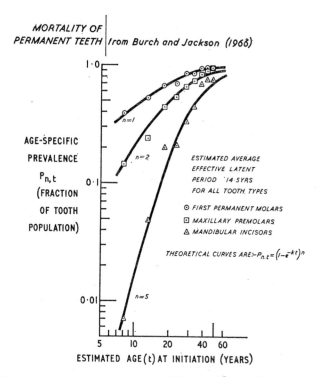

MORTALITY OF
PERMANENT TEETH (from Burch and Jackson (1968)

Fig. 3.2 Age-specific prevalence (P_t) of initiated disease (as a fraction of the *tooth* population), leading to the loss of permanent teeth, in relation to estimated age (t) at initiation (log–log scales). Latent period correction = 14.5 years throughout. From Burch and Jackson (1966a). The equation of the curve relating to first permanent molars is: $P_t = 1 - \exp(-kt)$, where the constant k is 0.054 yr^{-1}. Curves relating to maxillary premolar and mandibular incisor teeth are described in Chapter 4.

becomes mutant, it starts to propagate a forbidden-clone of descendant cells. The clonal cells synthesise autoantibodies, which then attack target cells bearing complementary antigens. At the end of the latent period, the severity of attack is sufficient to give rise to symptoms and/or signs of the disease.

If df forbidden-clones are initiated in a short time interval dt, we have:

$$df = Lm\,dt \qquad [3.11]$$

provided f_t, the average number of clones present at age t years is $\ll L$. This requires that mt should be $\ll 1$ for all t of interest. In other words, the mutation of a particular gene, in a particular cell, must be a *rare* as well as a random event. If $mt \ll 1$, then:

$$f_t = Lm\int_0^t dt = Lmt \qquad [3.12]$$

Writing k for Lm, which is the average gross mutation-rate per person, then the probability that a person will have at least one forbidden-clone at age t is given by:

$$1 - \exp(-kt) \qquad [3.13]$$

This probability that an individual will have at least one forbidden-clone at age t, is equal to the proportion of individuals of age t in the population with the initiated disease. That is, it is equal to the age-specific prevalence of the initiated disease, P_t. Hence,

$$P_t = 1 - \exp(-kt) \qquad [3.14]$$

This is the relation shown for first permanent molar teeth in Fig. 3.2, and given by equations [3.7] and [3.10].

Age-specific initiation-rates, dP/dt, are obtained by differentiating age-specific prevalence and hence:

$$dP/dt = k\exp(-kt) \qquad [3.15]$$

(Note a difference in the sign conventions between equations [3.5] and [3.15]. The decay of radioactive nuclei represents a *loss* from the population of initial atoms; the initiation of disease represents a *gain* to the population of diseased individuals.)

We could have constructed an even simpler model which would have yielded equations of the form [3.14] and [3.15], by assuming that each person has only one cell at mutational risk, rather than L cells. The population of individuals would then be equivalent to our radioactive source, which is a population of atoms. For biological reasons (see Chapter 9) I believe this is an over simplified model.

Many diseases (such as familial Mediterranean fever – Fig. 3.1) are confined to people with a particular form of inheritance. Suppose that people genetically predisposed to a particular disease constitute a fraction, S, of the general population. Also, suppose that S is effectively constant in time, and that age-specific mortality in the 'S sub-population' is the same as that in the general population; S will then be constant with age. If the disease is initiated by a single somatic mutation, of average gross-rate k per predisposed person, then the age-specific prevalence (P_t) of initiated disease with respect to the *general* population will be:

$$P_t = S\{1 - \exp(-kt)\} \qquad [3.16]$$

and the age-specific initiation rate (dP/dt) in the *general* population at age t will be:

$$dP/dt = k\,S \exp(-kt) \qquad [3.17]$$

The age-distributions of clinical dental caries in certain tooth types, and of grade 1 clinical inflammatory polyarthritis

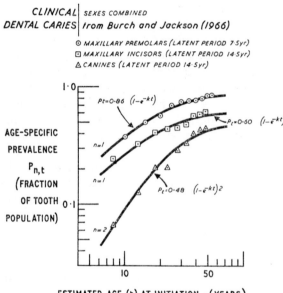

CLINICAL DENTAL CARIES | SEXES COMBINED / from Burch and Jackson (1966)

⊙ MAXILLARY PREMOLARS (LATENT PERIOD 7·5yr)
⊡ MAXILLARY INCISORS (LATENT PERIOD 14·5yr)
△ CANINES (LATENT PERIOD 14·5yr)

AGE-SPECIFIC PREVALENCE $P_{n,t}$ (FRACTION OF TOOTH POPULATION)

$P_t = 0.86 \ (1 - e^{-kt})$

$P_t = 0.60 \ (1 - e^{-kt})$

$P_t = 0.48 \ (1 - e^{-kt})^2$

ESTIMATED AGE (t) AT INITIATION (YEARS)

Fig. 3.3   Age-specific prevalence (P_t) of initiated disease (as a fraction of the *tooth* population) leading to clinical dental caries, in relation to estimated age (t) at initiation (log–log scales). From Burch and Jackson (1966a). Corrections have been applied for missing teeth. The equation referring to maxillary premolars is: $P_t = 0.86\{1 - \exp(-kt)\}$, and to maxillary incisors is: $P_t = 0.60\{1 - \exp(-kt)\}$. In both examples the value of k is 0·054 yr^{-1}. The equation of the curve describing the age-specific prevalance of caries in canine teeth is described in Chapter 4.

conform to the above equations [3.16] and [3.17] – see Fig. 3.3 and Burch (1966c).

In the next chapter and Chapters 9 and 11, we shall see that the age-distributions of many diseases follow more complicated statistics than those above. Nevertheless, in every example we shall consider – and in many more we shall not – the instability of any *particular* gene whose transition (mutation) contributes towards the initiation of a specific disease, can be described in terms of the fundamental differential equation [3.1] from birth, to all ages (*t*) of interest. More complicated age-patterns arise because *multiple* spontaneous gene changes are required to initiate the disease.

That the empirical law governing one important aspect of 'biological decay' in mammals has the same mathematical form as the law of radioactive decay is challenging: it hints at the underlying unity of physical, chemical, and at least some biological phenomena. No external event is needed to cause either the disintegration of the atomic nucleus, or, as I shall argue in the next three chapters, the gene transition. Nuclear disintegration arises from an intrinsic structural instability. Under normal physiological conditions in man (and probably in all mammals) it appears that the form of gene transition initiating many diseases depends only on the intrinsic instability of the macromolecular chemical complex. However, there is little doubt that abnormal factors, such as high levels of ionising radiation can induce such gene changes. The possible biochemical basis of spontaneous gene change will be discussed in Chapter 7.

PHILOSOPHIC TAILPIECE

Readers with a philosophic bent may like to contrast my broad conclusions concerning the nature of the mutational events in autoaggressive disease (see also the next four chapters) with Elsasser's (1966) very different assumptions concerning the fundamental properties of biological systems. Elsasser believes that every biological system is unique and that individuals form *inhomogeneous classes of finite membership*. To me, however, it appears that a specific mutational event, contributing to the initiation of a specific autoaggressive disease, can, like many physical and chemical phenomena, be ideally regarded as belonging to an *infinite homogeneous class*. As such, and according to von Neumann's (1955) theory, the frequency of occurrence of the mutational events should be deductively derivable from the laws of quantum mechanics. In Chapters 6 and 7, I reach the same conclusion by a different route.

4. THE SEX- AND AGE-DISTRIBUTIONS OF AUTOAGGRESSIVE DISEASE

'. . . to this day, our confidence in any science is roughly proportional to the amount of mathematics it employs—that is, to its ability to formulate its concepts with enough precision to allow them to be handled mathematically.'

J. Bronowski and B. Mazlish, 1963

Clinicians have long been aware that the sex- and age-distributions of many diseases are more-or-less the same from year to year, and from country to country. To take the example of Huntington's chorea it has been found that within large unselected series from the United States, Great Britain, Western Germany, and Australia, the numbers of male and female cases are almost equal, and the curve of age-specific onset-rates versus age is always bell-shaped, with a mode at about 40 years of age. Like Huntington's chorea, many other diseases with characteristic sex- and age-distributions, such as gout, psoriasis, and diabetes mellitus are known to be genetically-determined. Since the recognition of Garrod's work, many scientists have regarded such disorders as 'inborn errors of metabolism'. When inheritance is monogenic, the predisposing gene is supposed to produce a defective or deficient enzyme, and the symptoms and signs of disease are supposed to be traceable to a faulty or inadequate metabolism. To explain why such diseases are seldom manifested at birth, it is usually postulated that an environmental challenge – such as a dietary factor, a chance infection, or a situation producing mental stress – is necessary to evoke the pathological response which, hitherto, has been latent.

But if this explanation is correct, why should the age-distribution of the onset of such diseases be reproducible – at different times, and in different continents? It is inconceivable that the distribution and impact of dietary factors, infective agents, etc., could always be uniform from country to country, and from continent to continent. An insurmountable obstacle, in my view, is the detailed mathematical form of the sex- and age-patterns of such diseases: these reflect some quite general laws, one of which, concerning the nature of somatic gene instability, was mentioned in the previous chapter. Such laws cannot be reconciled with the notion of extrinsic initiating agents of the kind mentioned above.

Outside the cancer field, this eminently quantitative evidence relating to the sex- and age-distributions of disease has attracted little analytical attention. Ironically, it has been left to the non-mathematician Burnet (1965) to observe: 'If the form of age-incidence of a disease is reproducibly similar in different environments, this must be regarded as one of its characteristics and therefore calls for interpretation. Since it can be expressed graphically as a definite curve, it is susceptible to mathematical treatment and may therefore be relevant as evidence to test this or that hypothesis of aetiology.' Burnet (1965) regards the mathematical analysis of age patterns as '. . . a new and potentially powerful approach to an understanding of the aetiology of well-defined diseases of obscure origin'.

At the end of the last chapter I considered the age-distributions of diseases initiated by a single, random somatic mutation. We shall now proceed to the more general, and slightly more complicated case, of initiation by multiple somatic mutations.

DISEASE INITIATION BY MULTIPLE SOMATIC MUTATIONS

Analysis of the sex- and age-distributions of many diseases has shown that we need to examine three biological models, although a single mathematical formulation covers all three cases (Burch 1967a). Firstly, a single gene mutation, in each of several (n) cells, may be required to initiate the growth of multiple (n) forbidden-clones. The value of n can be at least as high as 5 in diseases such as the severe forms of clinical inflammatory polyarthritis, and the loss of certain permanent teeth – see Fig. 3.2 and Burch (1966c). In the second model, multiple (r) somatic mutations are required in a single stem cell, out of a population of similar cells at mutational risk, to trigger the growth of a single forbidden-clone. Usually, r is in the range 2 to 6, although it can, perhaps, be as high as 12

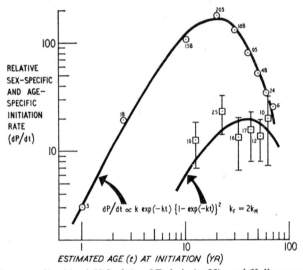

Fig. 4.1   Combined U.S. data of Dubois (1966), and Kellum and Haserick (1964), for 819 patients with systemic lupus erythematosus – see Burch and Rowell (1965a) for details. (This is often described as *the* autoimmune disease *par excellence*.) Theoretical curves are: $dP/dt \propto kS \exp(-kt)\{1 - \exp(-kt)\}^2$ where the k values are about 2.8×10^{-2} yr^{-1} (males), and 5.5×10^{-2} yr^{-1} (females). The ratio, S_F/S_M of predisposed females to males for the combined series is about 4.5. Latent period corrections are 5 years (females) and 2.5 years (males), except for the 0 to 4 years age range (females) where 1.5 years is assumed. The relatively poor fit of the initiation-rates for males to the theoretical curve may reflect in part the diagnostic difficulties connected with this complex disease. However, the numbers of male patients are small, and an indication of approximate statistical errors is shown. Bars on the error limits are calculated from: $n \pm 2\sqrt{n}$, where n is the number of cases.

(see Fig. 4.15). Occasionally, a third model is implicated, in which the disease is initiated by multiple (n) forbidden-clones, where each clone derives from a stem cell in which multiple (r) somatic mutations have occurred. (See Figs 4.13, 11.6 and 11.11; also Burch 1968b.)

Consider the first model in more detail, and suppose a particular disease is confined to a genetically-specific sub-

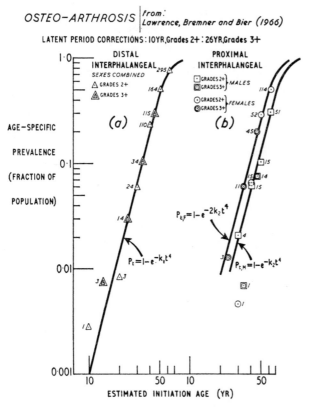

Fig. 4.2 Age-specific prevalence for osteo-arthrosis of: (a) distal interphalangeal joints; (b) proximal interphalangeal joints. From Leigh and Wensleydale survey by Lawrence *et al.* (1966). There are no systematic sex-differences in the data for interphalangeal joints. In (b), the value of k_2 for females is double that for males, indicating that one of the four random initiating events is X-linked. Common latent period corrections (10 years for grade 2+, and 26 years for grade 3+) have been applied to all the data. Hence the average time involved in progressing from a grade 2 to a grade 3 lesion is 16 years. About 100 per cent of the Leigh and Wensleydale populations ($S = 1$) are predisposed to osteo-arthrosis in one or more of these joints. The value of k_1 is about 9×10^{-8} yr^{-4}, and that of k_2 is about 2.5×10^{-8} yr^{-4}. (Taken from Burch (1968b).)

population which constitutes a fraction, S, of the general population at birth. Each predisposed person has n phenotypically distinctive sets of cells at mutational risk, and each set consists of a population of L cells. (Mutations and other 'errors' apart, all normal diploid cells in an individual are

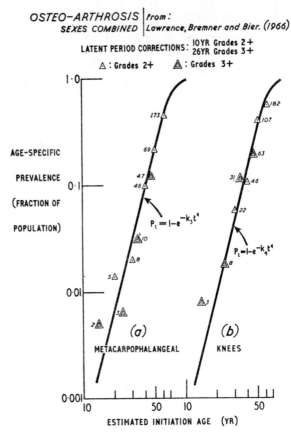

Fig. 4.3 Similar findings to those in Fig. 4.2 but for: (a) meta-carpophalangeal, and (b) knee joints (Lawrence *et al.* 1966). There are no systematic sex-differences in these data. The same latent period corrections have been applied as in Fig. 4.2. The value of k_3 is about 4×10^{-8} yr^{-4}, and of k_4 about 6×10^{-8} yr^{-4}. From the excellent internal consistency of these data, and their striking agreement with autoaggressive statistics, we can conclude that the rate of progression of osteo-arthrosis in all four types of joint is remarkably uniform. (Taken from Burch (1968b).)

genetically identical – because they descend from the common zygote – but the genes that *function* differ from cell type to cell type according to biochemical, immunological, and morpho-logical differentiation (see Chapters 6 and 9).) We postulate that the disease will be initiated when at least one cell has become mutant, in each of the *n* sets of cells. All possible sequences of events are equally effective. The average rate of mutation, in each cell at risk, is m per *unit time*, and we define the gross somatic mutation-rate per set – that is, Lm – as being equal to k.

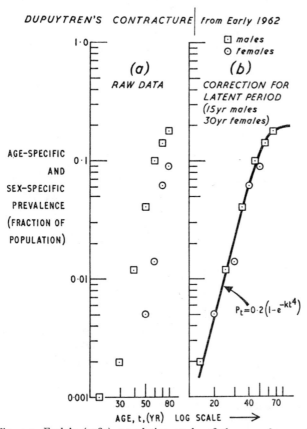

Fig. 4.4 Early's (1962) population study of the prevalence of Dupuytren's contracture. When latent period corrections are applied to the raw data in (a) – 15 years for men, 30 years for women – the corrected points for both sexes fit the common theoretical curve: $P = 0.2\{1 - \exp(-kt^4)\}$, with $k \simeq 1.7 \times 10^{-7}$ yr^{-4}. (Taken from Burch (1966a).)

(As before we require $mt \ll 1$.) If k is constant from birth to the onset of disease, and constant with respect to time, then we saw in the previous chapter that the probability that at least one initiating somatic mutation will have occurred, in one set of cells, in a predisposed person by age t is: $\{1 - \exp(-kt)\}$.

Because the initiating somatic mutations are random and independent of one another, the probability that at least one mutation will have occurred in each of the n sets of L cells in a predisposed person by age t, will be: $\{1 - \exp(-kt)\}^n$. Provided

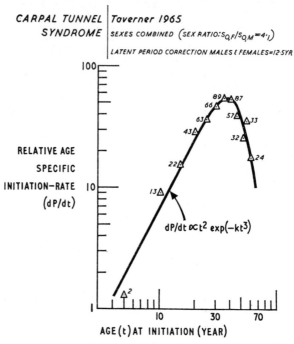

Fig. 4.5 Taverner's (1965) data for carpal tunnel syndrome. The sex-ratio S_F/S_M of predisposed females to males is about 4·1. Other parameters are the same for both sexes and the data have been combined. These parameters are $r = 3$; $k \simeq 1\cdot3 \times 10^{-5}\ \mathrm{yr}^{-3}$; $\lambda = 12\cdot5$ yr. Predisposition will be polygenic involving sex-linked and autosomal factors. (Taken from Burch (1966c).)

S does not change appreciably with time, and provided age-specific mortality-rates in the predisposed and general populations are similar, then the age-specific prevalence (P_t) of the initiated disease in the overall population will be given by:

$$P_t = S\{1 - \exp(-kt)\}^n \qquad [4.1]$$

(More generally, if the k values for each distinctive forbidden-clone are $k_1, k_2, \ldots, k_n$ respectively, then:

$$P_t = S\left[\{1 - \exp(-k_1 t)\}\{1 - \exp(-k_2 t)\} \ldots \{1 - \exp(-k_n t)\}\right] \qquad [4.2]$$

Figs. 3.2 and 3.3 show examples of age-distributions conforming to equation [4.1], where values of n range from 1 to 5. Equation [4.1] is an example of the Yule, or homogeneous-birth process.

Age-specific initiation-rates (dP/dt) for the model described by equation [4.1] can be obtained by differentiation:

$$dP/dt = nkS \exp(-kt)\{1 - \exp(-kt)\}^{n-1} \qquad [4.3]$$

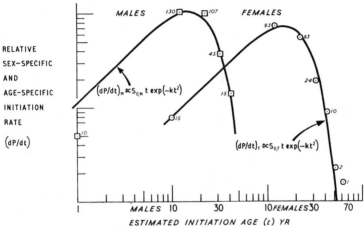

WILSON'S DISEASE | O'Reilly 1967

LATENT PERIOD CORRECTION=4YEARS (both sexes) $S_{0M}/S_{0F}=1\cdot4$

Fig. 4.6   O'Reilly's (1967) data for Wilson's disease. The sex-ratio $S_M/S_F \simeq 1\cdot4$; $r = 2$; $k \simeq 2\cdot2 \times 10^{-3}$ yr^{-2} (both sexes); and the latent period correction is 4 years. Genetic predisposition will involve sex-linked as well as autosomal factors.

Fig. 4.1 shows an example of an age-distribution fitting equation [4.3] where the value of n is 3. (See also Fig. 11.9.) Age-specific onset-rates, from which age-specific initiation-raset can usually be readily derived, have one advantage over age-specific prevalence. For their interpretation they require that age-specific mortality-rates in the predisposed population, should be approximately equal to those in the general population, only up to the age of onset of the disease in question. Thus they can be used in the study of fatal diseases. Age-specific onset-rates have the additional advantage that they contain more 'structure' and they enable age-patterns to be analysed

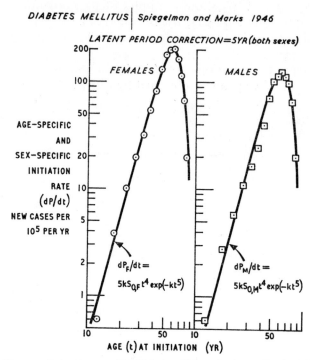

Fig. 4·7   Spiegelman and Marks's (1946) data for the predominantly late onset form of diabetes mellitus. The statistical parameters are: $r = 5$; $S_F \simeq 6.7 \times 10^{-2}$; $S_M \simeq 4 \times 10^{-2}$; and $k_F = k_M \simeq 1.0 \times 10^{-9} \mathrm{yr}^{-5}$. Often regarded as an autosomal recessive disorder, a sex-linked factor – probably a dominant-effect X-linked allele of frequency 0·33 (in this U.S. population) – is also implicated (Burch 1966c). It follows that the frequency of the autosomal contribution in this population is 0·12; if 'recessive', the frequency of the predisposing autosomal allele is nearly 0·35. An early onset form of diabetes mellitus (with $r = 2$, and an initiation mode at about 10 years) is found in which more males are predisposed than females (Westlund 1966).

from relatively small numbers of cases more accurately than is possible from comparable age-specific prevalence data.

The second model involving multiple random initiating events – r somatic mutations in a single stem cell – fits the age-distributions for many diseases. Suppose that L stem cells are at somatic mutational risk in a predisposed person, and that r specific mutations (each of average rate m, per gene at risk, per cell at risk, per year), are required in any one stem cell to initiate the disease. Assuming $mt \ll 1$, and adopting the usual provisos concerning S, it can readily be shown (Burch 1965, 1966b) that the age-specific prevalence (P_t) of initiated disease will be described by:

$$P_t = S\{1 - \exp(-kt^r)\} \qquad [4.4]$$

Here, k is defined as Lm^r. (More generally, if the mutation-

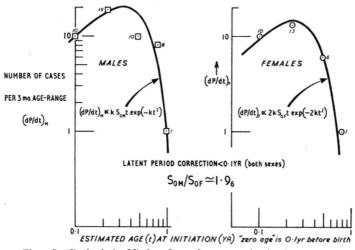

Fig. 4.8   Caplan's (1966) data for early onset urticaria pigmentosa. An interesting example of a disease, presumably autoaggressive, in which there is almost complete penetrance in one genotype before the end of the first year of postnatal life. No fundamental distinction can be drawn between the pathogenesis of this disease and that of many ageing conditions. 'Zero age' on the time-scale is taken to be 0·1 yr prior to birth. Other parameters are: $r = 2$; $S_M/S_F \simeq 1.96$; $k_F \simeq 9.4 \text{ yr}^{-2}$; $k_M \simeq 4.7 \text{ yr}^{-2}$; $\lambda < 0.1$ yr.

rates of individual genes are $m_1, m_2, \ldots, m_r$ respectively, then $k = Lm_1 . m_2 \ldots m_r$.) Figs 4.2 to 4.4 show age-distributions conforming to equation [4.4].

Differentiating equation [4.4] to obtain age-specific initiation rates, we have:

$$dP/dt = rkSt^{(r-1)} \exp(-kt^r) \qquad [4.5]$$

These last two equations are versions of the Weibull renewal process. Many diseases conform to equation [4.5] as can be seen from Figs 4.5 to 4.12, and other examples in Chapters 9 and 11. Ashley (1967) has shown that the age-distribution of acute appendicitis fits equation [4.5] with $r = 2$.

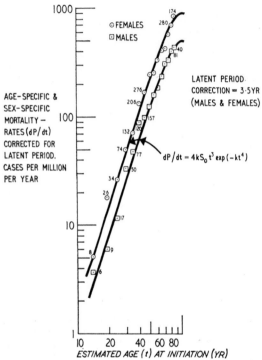

MORTALITY FROM DISEASES OF MITRAL VALVE
ENGLAND AND WALES

(CATEGORIES 410 AND 421·0 INTERNATIONAL STATISTICAL
CLASSIFICATION)

FROM: REGISTRAR GENERAL'S STATISTICAL REVIEW FOR YEAR 1961

Fig. 4.9 Whereas the age-patterns illustrated hitherto have referred to chronic, and generally non-lethal conditions, this example of diseases of the mitral valve is taken from mortality statistics (Registrar General 1963). The parameters of the curves are: $r = 4$; $S_F = 6·4 \times 10^{-2}$; $S_M = 3·5 \times 10^{-2}$; $k_F = k_M \simeq 7·5 \times 10^{-9}$ yr^{-4}; $\lambda_F = \lambda_M = 3·5$ yr.

In the third model, where each of the n phenotypically-distinctive forbidden-clones is initiated by r somatic mutations, in a single stem cell, we simply combine equations [4.1] and [4.4]:

$$P_t = S\{1 - \exp(-kt^r)\}^n \qquad [4.6]$$

Age-specific initiation-rates (dP/dt) are obtained by differentiating the above equation for age-specific prevalence:

$$dP/dt = nrkSt^{(r-1)} \exp(-kt^r)\{1 - \exp(-kt)^r\}^{n-1} \qquad [4.7]$$

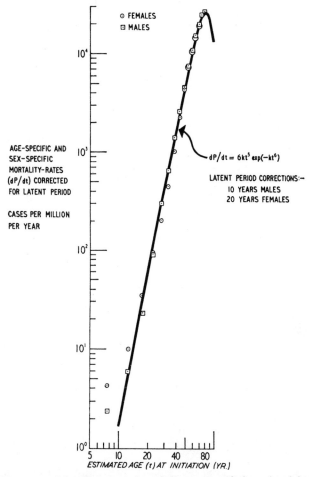

MORTALITY FROM HEART DISEASE SPECIFIED AS INVOLVING CORONARY ARTERIES ENGLAND AND WALES

(CATEGORY 420·1. INTERNATIONAL STATISTICAL CLASSIFICATION)

FROM: REGISTRAR GENERAL'S STATISTICAL REVIEW FOR YEAR 1961

⊙ FEMALES
▣ MALES

AGE-SPECIFIC AND
SEX-SPECIFIC
MORTALITY-RATES
(dP/dt) CORRECTED
FOR LATENT PERIOD

CASES PER MILLION
PER YEAR

$dP/dt = 6kt^5 \exp(-kt^6)$

LATENT PERIOD CORRECTIONS:—
10 YEARS MALES
20 YEARS FEMALES

ESTIMATED AGE (t) AT INITIATION (YR.)

Fig. 4.10 Mortality from heart disease specified as involving coronary arteries – category 420.1 (Registrar General 1963). This is the most important single cause of death in England and Wales—Parameters are: $r = 6$; $S_F = S_M \simeq 1$; $k_F = k_M \simeq 3·2 \times 10^{-12}$ yr^{-6}; $\lambda_F = 20$ years; $\lambda_M = 10$ years. Discrepancies below $t = 15$ years may represent diagnostic errors, and/or errors in the latent period correction, and/or a small contribution from one or more genotypes with predominantly early onset. A high average lifespan requires that the common lethal diseases should be characterised by a high value of r.

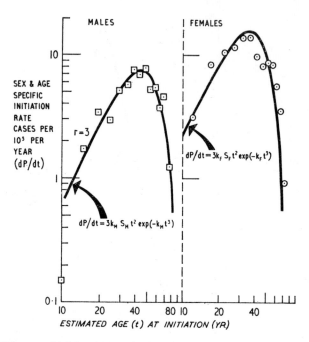

MANIC DEPRESSIVE PSYCHOSIS
NEW YORK STATE 1949–1951 (MALZBERG 1955)

Fig. 4.11   Malzberg's (1955) data for admissions to hospital in New York State, 1949 to 1951, with the diagnosis of manic depressive psychosis. Diagnostic difficulties complicate the interpretation of the statistics of psychoses. In 1949 to 1951 age-patterns indicate that some women with schizophrenia, and others with involutional psychoses, are still being classified as manic depressives. Earlier statistics, both for men and women (for details see Burch 1964a,b,c), show these tendencies in a much more exaggerated form. Curves are represented by the following parameters: $r = 3$; $S_F \simeq 5.7 \times 10^{-3}$; $S_M \simeq 3.4 \times 10^{-3}$; $k_F \simeq 1.4 \times 10^{-5} \text{ yr}^{-3}$; $k_M \simeq 7 \times 10^{-6} \text{ yr}^{-3}$; $\lambda_F = 5$ years; $\lambda_M = 2.5$ years. For the genetic analysis of the familial evidence, see Burch (1964a).

In a mathematical sense, this third model includes the first two. On putting $r = 1$, we obtain equations [4.1] and [4.3], and on putting $n = 1$, we obtain equation [4.4] and [4.5]. Hence, the general equations [4.6] and [4.7] describe the age-distributions of all the diseases we shall consider in this book – and of many more besides. Very often – but not always –

either n, or r, is equal to unity. Fig. 4.13 shows an example of a disease, involutional psychosis, where $n = 3$ and $r = 4$ (see also Figs 11.6 and 11.11).

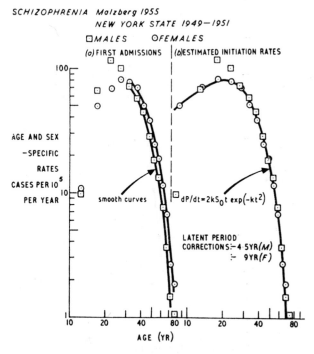

Fig. 4.12 Malzberg's (1955) data for admissions to hospital in New York State, 1949 to 1951, with the diagnosis of schizophrenia. Parameters describing the age pattern are: $r = 2$; $k \simeq 1 \cdot 25 \times 10^{-3}$ yr^{-2}; $S \simeq 2 \cdot 7 \times 10^{-2}$; $\lambda_{\mathrm{F}} = 9$ years; $\lambda_{\mathrm{M}} = 4 \cdot 5$ years. (See Burch (1964b) for the genetic analysis of familial evidence.) The departure of three of the points for males from the theoretical curve (an under-shoot followed by an overshoot) probably reflects an initial reluctance to diagnose schizophrenia in the young potential breadwinner, followed by a delayed admission to hospital.

That the age-patterns of so many diseases should conform so accurately to a single general differential equation is astonishing. So far as I am aware no one has ever anticipated the existence of such a widespread law in this notoriously unpredictable field of pathology.

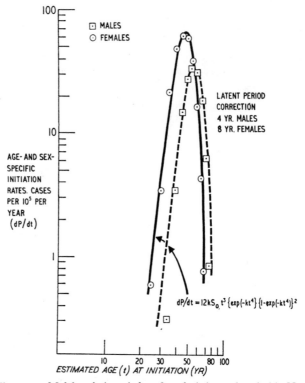

INVOLUTIONAL PSYCHOSES
NEW YORK STATE 1949–1951 (FROM: MALZBERG 1955)

☐ MALES
○ FEMALES

LATENT PERIOD
CORRECTION
4 YR. MALES
8 YR. FEMALES

AGE- AND SEX-
SPECIFIC
INITIATION
RATES. CASES
PER 10^5 PER
YEAR
(dP/dt)

$dP/dt = 12kS_0\, t^3 \{exp(-kt^4)\}\{1\text{-}exp(-kt^4)\}^2$

ESTIMATED AGE (t) AT INITIATION (YR)

Fig. 4.13   Malzberg's (1955) data for admission to hospital in New York State, 1949 to 1951, with the diagnosis of involutional psychosis. Parameters describing the age pattern are: $n = 3$; $r = 4$; $k_F \simeq 3 \cdot 2 \times 10^{-7}$ yr^{-4}; $k_M \simeq 1 \cdot 6 \times 10^{-7}$ yr^{-4}; $S_F \simeq 1 \cdot 24 \times 10^{-2}$; $S_M \simeq 7 \cdot 6 \times 10^{-3}$; $\lambda_F = 8$ years; $\lambda_M = 4$ years. A genetic scheme has been derived from the familial evidence (Burch 1964c).

USE OF LOG–LOG SCALES

When plotted on log–log graph paper the above mathematical functions have some very convenient properties. For a given size of grid, the curves for particular n and/or r values, *always retain the same shape,* for all values of k and of S. Plotting age (t) on the abscissa, the value of k affects the left-right location of the curve; high k values produce a shift to the left (towards

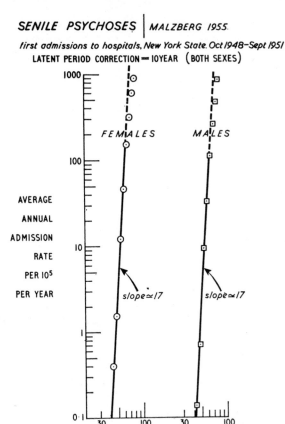

SENILE PSYCHOSES | *MALZBERG 1955.*

first admissions to hospitals, New York State. Oct 1948–Sept 1951
LATENT PERIOD CORRECTION — 10 YEAR (BOTH SEXES)

FEMALES   MALES

AVERAGE
ANNUAL
ADMISSION
RATE
PER 10^5
PER YEAR

slope ≈ 17   slope ≈ 17

ESTIMATED AGE (t) AT INITIATION (YR)

Fig. 4.14   Malzberg's (1955) statistics for senile psychoses in New York State 1948 to 1951. These show an exceptionally steep dependence on age. Because there is little departure from a simple power law, even at the end of the lifespan, the details of n and/or r cannot be deduced mathematically. Probably 18 random initiating events are required.

low t). S affects the up and down position of the curve. Accordingly, each function, for discrete values of n and/or r, can be drawn on tracing paper, and then, maintaining horizontal-vertical alignment, it can be superimposed on the raw data plotted on the log–log graph paper.

Every one of the above equations [4.1] to [4.7] becomes a simple power function when kt is appreciably less than unity,

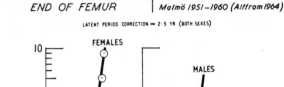

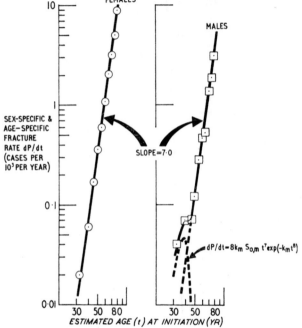

Fig. 4.15 Alffram's (1964) data for fractures at the proximal end (cervical region) of the femur. Regarded as a typical ageing condition. The age-specific fracture-rate for women is quite accurately proportional to the seventh power of age from 30 to 80 years. If the data for younger men are confirmed, they will indicate the existence of of a distinctive group, genetically predisposed to early-onset cervical fractures of the femur.

and hence they all become straight lines on a log–log graph at low kt. Age-distributions following a simple power law over a substantial part of the lifespan are shown in Figs 4.14 to 4.16. (Differences in the sex- and age-distributions of cervical fractures of the femur (Fig. 4.15), trochanteric fractures of the femur (Fig. 4.16), and fractures of the distal forearm (Fig. 4.17) reflect marked differences in pathogenetic mechanisms. It follows that fractures are not the simple consequences of a uniform and generalised osteoporotic process.)

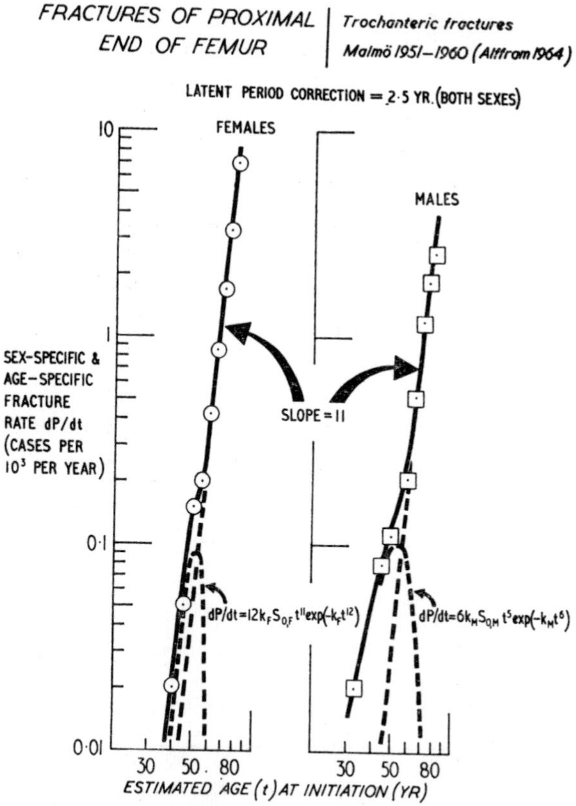

Fig. 4.16 Alffram's (1964) data for trochanteric fractures of the femur. Despite the proximity of the cervical and trochanteric fracture regions, the age-distributions here are much steeper than in Fig. 4.15. Different forbidden-clones, with different target cells are implicated. (The remarkable anatomical specificity of autoaggressive disorders is discussed in Chapter 8.) These important data indicate that the value of r can sometimes be as high as 12. They also suggest that early onset trochanteric fractures are mainly confined to distinctive genotypes.

Taking the special case: $n = 1$ and $r = 1$, and substituting in equation [4.7], we have: $dP/dt = S \exp(-kt)$, and hence $\ln(dP/dt) = \ln S - kt$. As pointed out in Chapter 3, when we plot $\ln(dP/dt)$ against t on a linear scale, we obtain a straight line for all values of t that are of interest. For this special function, it is therefore preferable to use semi-logarithmic graph paper, plotting dP/dt on the logarithmic scale, and t on the linear one.

In the log–log graph of equation [4.1], the slope of the straight line at low kt is n; for equation [4.3] it is $(n-1)$; for equation [4.4] it is r; for [4.5] it is $(r-1)$; for [4.6] it is nr; and for [4.7] it is $(nr-1)$. As kt approaches unity, the power law dependence of P, and of dP/dt on t, is no longer maintained, and the slope of the curve decreases. For equal n and r values,

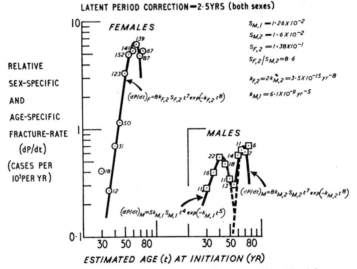

Fig. 4.17   Alffram's (1964) data for first fracture of the distal forearm. Further emphasis is given to the specificity of autoaggressive disease. Although trauma may often precipitate this type of fracture, the regularities in the statistics, and their close conformity to our theoretical equations indicate that the underlying pathogenesis of the condition is generally autoaggressive. For early onset male cases: $r = 5$; $S \simeq 1.3 \times 10^{-2}$; $k \simeq 6 \times 10^{-9}$ yr^{-5}. For most female, and for late onset male cases: $r = 8$; $S_F \simeq 0.138$; $S_M \simeq 1.6 \times 10^{-2}$; $k_F \simeq 3.5$ $10 \times^{-15}$ yr^{-8}; $k_M \simeq 1.75 \times 10^{-15}$ yr^{-8}.

equation [4.1] gives a more gradual shoulder than [4.4], but equations [4.1], [4.4], and [4.6] always approach the value S asymptotically if kt becomes appreciably greater than unity. In the differential forms, the slope of dP/dt versus t becomes zero at the modal initiation age, and then increasingly negative with increasing t. For the same values of n and of r, equation [4.3] gives a broader curve (see Fig. 4.1 with $n = 3$), than equation [4.5], (see Fig. 4.5 with $r = 3$).

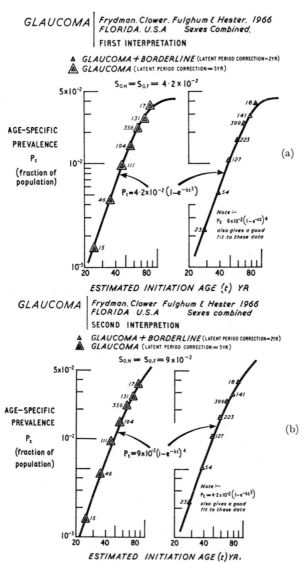

GLAUCOMA | Frydman. Clower. Fulghum & Hester. 1966
FLORIDA. U.S.A   Sexes Combined.

FIRST INTERPRETATION

▲ GLAUCOMA + BORDERLINE (LATENT PERIOD CORRECTION = 2YR)
▲ GLAUCOMA (LATENT PERIOD CORRECTION = 5YR)

$S_{0,M} = S_{0,F} = 4.2 \times 10^{-2}$

AGE-SPECIFIC
PREVALENCE
P_t
(fraction of
population)

(a)

$P_t = 4.2 \times 10^{-2} (1 - e^{-kt^3})$

Note :—
$P_t \quad 9 \times 10^{-2} (1 - e^{-ct})^4$
also gives a good
fit to these data

ESTIMATED INITIATION AGE (t) YR

GLAUCOMA | Frydman. Clower Fulghum & Hester 1966
FLORIDA U.S.A   Sexes combined

SECOND INTERPRETION

▲ GLAUCOMA + BORDERLINE (LATENT PERIOD CORRECTION = 2YR)
▲ GLAUCOMA (LATENT PERIOD CORRECTION = 5YR)

$S_{0,M} = S_{0,F} = 9 \times 10^{-2}$

AGE-SPECIFIC
PREVALENCE
P_t
(fraction of
population)

(b)

$P_t = 9 \times 10^{-2} (1 - e^{-kt})^4$

Note :—
$P_t = 4.2 \times 10^{-2} (1 - e^{-kt^3})$
also gives a good
fit to these data

ESTIMATED INITIATION AGE (t) YR.

Fig. 4.18a and b. Illustrating possible ambiguities of interpretation. Population study of the prevalence of glaucoma (Frydman
et al. 1966). A slightly better fit is given by $P = 9 \times 10^{-2}\{1 - \exp
(-kt)\}^4$, than by Weibull statistics, but more extensive data,
covering a still wider age range, are needed for confirmation. If
Yule statistics (Fig. 4.17b) are relevant $k \simeq 1.6 \times 10^{-2}\,\mathrm{yr}^{-1}$, and 9
per cent of the population studied are at risk. On either interpreta-
tion, the disease would appear to be autoagressive, and the average
time taken to deteriorate from the diagnostic categories 'borderline'
to definite glaucoma is 3 years, regardless of sex and age at onset.

Taken over a *sufficiently wide range* of kt, the shape of every curve for a distinctive n and/or r is unique, and the figures illustrated have been selected to demonstrate their different characteristics. However, when the t range of the observations is limited, ambiguities of interpretation can arise, and one such example is shown in Figs 4.18 a and b.

CURVE-FITTING

Given suitable and unbiased raw data, only one adjustment is permissible when carrying out curve-fitting – the application of a correction for latent period. When we examine the age-prevalence of Dupuytren's contracture (Fig. 4.4), age-specific hospital admission-rates for schizophrenia (Fig. 4.12), and age-specific mortality-rates for coronary artery disease (Fig. 4.10), we find that the uncorrected age-patterns are similar for the two sexes, but that the curve for females lags behind the curve for males. For a given population, this time lag is effectively constant at all ages above about 10 years, and it indicates that the difference in the average latent periods for the two sexes $(\lambda_F - \lambda_M)$ is approximately constant throughout most of life. We find that when we put $\lambda_M = \lambda_F - \lambda_M$ (and therefore, $\lambda_F = 2\lambda_M$), and when we apply these constant latent period corrections to the raw data, then the adjusted points, for both males and females, fit one version of our standard stochastic equations (see Figs 4.4 and 4.12).

We find a similar situation in connection with certain diseases such as osteo-arthrosis (Figs 4.2 and 4.3) and glaucoma (Figs 4.18 a and b), where the clinical severity can be graded, and where, for example, clinical grade 3 osteo-arthrosis follows grade 2 after an average interval of about 16 years, regardless of the joints examined, and regardless of age. This implies that the average rate of progression of this disease, from grade 2 to grade 3, is independent of the age of initiation – at least in adults. Application of a latent period correction of 10 years to grade 2+ (that is, grades 2 and above) and of 26 years to grade 3+, causes the corrected data for both grades to lie on the theoretical curve: $P_t = 1 - \exp(-kt^4)$.

When these simple sex-differences or grade-differences are absent, we have to adopt a trial-and-error procedure to correct for latent period. Suppose we have age-specific onset-rates by quinquennial age-groups: 10 to 14, 15 to 19, 20 to 24 years, etc. These can generally be approximated, with only small errors, to onset-rates at the instantaneous ages of 12·5, 17·5, 22·5 years, etc. If these data are now plotted at say 10·5, 15·5 and 20·5 years, etc., we have applied a 'latent period correction' of 2·0 years, and we can compare the graphed points with our standard curves drawn on tracing paper. If the fit to a standard curve is satisfactory at all ages we need proceed no further, but if there is a systematic and increasing divergence between the plotted points and the nearest standard curve as we proceed from high t down to low t, then the latent period correction is either too large or too small. (The latent period correction has only a small effect on the shape of the curve at high t, but a pronounced effect at low t.) If at low t the adjusted data points fall below the theoretical curve, the applied correction is too small; if above, it is too large. With some practice, a good fit can usually be obtained between statistically and diagnostically reliable data for a spontaneous autoaggressive disease, and a standard curve at the second trial – provided the disease is genetically homogeneous.

Fully rigorous curve-fitting would require a knowledge of the *distribution* of the latent period, and preferably, very narrow age-ranges. The methods described above make the implicit assumption that the latent period for a given disease, in a given population, is the same for all individuals of a given sex. In a perfectly uniform environment, and in the absence of stress, we might expect the latent period distribution to be governed only by the growth and progression of the forbidden-clone. For a given genotype, the distribution should then be narrow, approaching a delta function. However, the data show that environmental factors can modify the duration of the latent period (see Figs 4.20 a and b and 4.21 a to g), and it follows that the distribution of the latent period will be broadened. In general, its shape will differ from one environment to another. So far, there is no direct method for determining the overall latent period distribution in man (we cannot observe initiation) and hence fully rigorous curve-fitting is not possible. However, in age-distribution analysis we aim to establish the basic pathogenesis of disease, and for this purpose, the approximate method of analysis is usually adequate. An error of, say, $\pm$ 10 per cent in the average latent period is not very important at this stage of our inquiry.

A biological complication intrudes, however, during the early years. An important part of the delay between the initiation and the onset of autoaggressive disease, is evidently due to the action of an endogenous defence mechanism which is directed against forbidden-clones (see Chapter 9). This defence is probably mediated through immunoglobulins. The cell system that synthesizes immunoglobulins is not fully developed at birth, and most IgG immunoglobulins present in the newborn, and for some months after, are of maternal origin. Accordingly, the average latent period during the infant and early childhood years is expected to be shorter than in adults: the evidence supports this expectation (Burch and Rowell 1965a; Burch 1966c).

I have deliberately stressed the (generally slight) limitations of curve-fitting, although examination of the figures will show that the agreement between the simply adjusted data and theory is often most impressive. The high measure of agreement between data collected from different clinical series, often from different countries, is especially noteworthy. (See Figs 4.21 a to g, 11.1, 11.2, 11.4, 11.5; Burch 1968a; Burch and Rowell 1968.)

SEX DIFFERENCES

Analysis of the sex- and age-distributions shows that, for a given disease, the values for S, and/or k, and /or λ, may differ as between men and women.

The parameter S defines the proportion of the population that is predisposed to the disease. Whenever adequate familial and twins evidence has been available, it has shown that predisposition is determined by genetic factors (Burch 1964a,b,c, 1966a, 1968a; Burch and Rowell 1965a,b). Consequently, sex differences in S should generally be attributed either to predisposing X and/or Y-linked genes, or to cytoplasmic inheritance. In many diseases, it appears that X-linkage is involved, although I predict that Y-linkage will be found to be associated with others. However, even when S shows a sex-difference, the particular n and/or r values in the equations which describe the age-distributions in the two sexes, are nearly always the same. Nevertheless, the value of k may then differ between the sexes, and when it does, I have always found $k_F = 2k_M$. This implies that the average rate of certain initiating events is twice as high in females as in males. Under these circumstances the initiation mode occurs earlier in the female population than in the male one. Very occasionally, as with gout, the *form* of the age patterns in the two sexes is different (Burch 1968b). In such situations we must suspect the participation of Y-linked factors, either in the predisposing male genotype, and/or in the initiating events in males. Pertinently, gout is often transmitted through the paternal line to sons (Dixon 1968), and this supports Y-linkage, although X-linkage is not ruled out as an additional factor: autosomal factors are almost certainly implicated as well (Burch 1968b).

Only one type of sex-difference in the latent period (λ) is common: $\lambda_F = 2\lambda_M$. This differential is discussed below.

KARYOTYPIC ABNORMALITIES

Individuals with Down's syndrome usually possess three, instead of the normal pair of chromosomes 21. (It is still not completely certain, however, whether chromosome 22, and not 21 is involved.) Acute leukaemia is much more common in Down's syndrome than in the general population, and differences in the age patterns for childhood leukaemia are also observed. These show that the k values in Down's patients are higher, and this immensely important feature is discussed in Chapter 11.

GENETIC HETEROGENEITY

Some diseases which appear to be more-or-less homogeneous by ordinary diagnostic criteria show two, or even three age-onset modes within the same sex (see Figs 4.15 to 4.17, 4.19 to 4.22, and other examples in Chapters 9 and 11). When two (or three) versions of stochastic equation [4.7] are required to fit the overall age-distribution, I conclude that two (or three) genetically-distinctive sub-populations are predisposed

5

to the disease, and that the onset-pattern in each sub population is characteristic of that group.

Significantly, detailed clinical studies confirm the indications of heterogeneity given by the analysis of age distributions. In

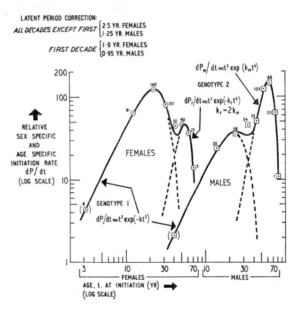

Fig. 4.19 Data of Howard *et al.* (1965) for myasthenia gravis, which is widely regarded as a classical 'autoimmune' disease. The closeness of fit to autoaggressive statistics is certainly striking. The bimodal age-pattern reveals two genetically-distinctive forms of the disease. Females predominate among early onset cases, whereas most late onset cases are men. For the early onset group (genotype 1): $r = 3$; $S_F/S_M \simeq 3.4$; $k_F = k_M \simeq 5.9 \times 10^{-5}$ yr^{-3}. For genotype 2: $r = 6$; $S_M/S_F \simeq 3.5$; $k_F \simeq 3.5 \times 10^{-11}$ yr^{-6}; $k_M \simeq 1.75 \times 10^{-11}$ yr^{-6}. In both genotypes, the latent period in females (λ_F) is double that of males (λ_M). (From Burch 1966c.)

Huntington's chorea, the age patterns of the distinguishable clinical forms of the disease are described by different versions of equation [4.5] (Burch 1968a). From the sex- and age-distributions of psoriasis we predicted (Burch and Rowell 1965b) that the early and late onset forms would be found to be genetically-distinctive, and Farber and Carlsen (1966)

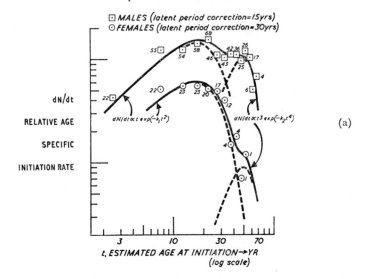

DUODENAL ULCER | RURAL YORK. 1952–1962

□ MALES (latent period correction=15yrs)
⊙ FEMALES (latent period correction=30yrs)

dN/dt

RELATIVE AGE

SPECIFIC

INITIATION RATE

$dN/dt \propto t\, exp(-k_1 t^2)$

$dN/dt \propto t^3 exp(-k_2 t^4)$

(a)

t, ESTIMATED AGE AT INITIATION→YR
(log scale)

3   10   30   70

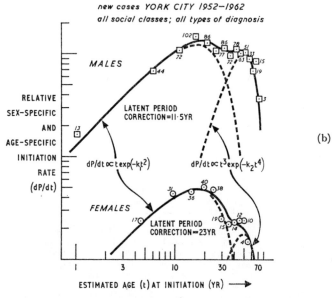

DUODENAL ULCER   Pulvertaft 1965
new cases YORK CITY 1952–1962
all social classes; all types of diagnosis

MALES

RELATIVE
SEX-SPECIFIC
AND
AGE-SPECIFIC
INITIATION
RATE
(dP/dt)

LATENT PERIOD
CORRECTION=11·5YR

$dP/dt \propto t\, exp(-k_1 t^2)$

$dP/dt \propto t^3 exp(-k_2 t^4)$

FEMALES

LATENT PERIOD
CORRECTION=23YR

(b)

1   3   10   30   70

ESTIMATED AGE (t) AT INITIATION (YR) ——▶

Fig. 4.20

(see caption on p. 60)

have since shown that these two groups are in fact genetically and clinically distinctive. Whereas the childhood group has 52 per cent of relatives with psoriasis; the corresponding figure for the adult group is 30 per cent. Clinical differences have been predicted and confirmed with respect to ulcerative colitis: late onset cases prove to have a generally milder form of the disease than early onset cases (Edwards and Truelove 1963; de Dombal 1967a). Deductions concerning genetic hetero-geneity made from age-pattern analysis are therefore verified by careful clinical and familial studies.

Before embarking on the genetic analysis of diseases, the sex- and age-specific patterns of their onset or prevalence must first be examined. In this way, the minimum number of genetically-distinctive sub-populations predisposed to the disease can usually be assessed, and when absolute onset-rates (or prevalences for chronic diseases) are available, S can be calculated for each sex, and for each genotype, separately. The value of S is needed to determine the frequency of predisposing genes.

Fig. 4.20 a and b (*on p. 59*). Pulvertaft's (1965) data for York city, and rural York patients, with duodenal ulcer (first attack) during the years 1952 to 1962 inclusive (see Burch 1966c). Duodenal ulcer is not generally regarded as an autoaggressive disease, although Pulvertaft's statistics, the histopathology (Magnus 1962) and the clinical course (Jennings 1965) are highly consistent with this interpretation. Mackay and Hislop (1966) have independently put forward an 'autoimmune' interpretation based on histopathological studies. Two distinctive genotypes are apparent, and the age-patterns are described by: $r = 2$; $k \simeq 2 \cdot 0 \times 10^{-3}$ yr^{-2} for early onset cases; and $r = 4$; $k \simeq 1 \cdot 2 \times 10^{-7}$ yr^{-4} for late onset cases. One of the most interesting features of these statistics is the urban-rural difference in latent periods. For York city, latent period corrections (λ) are 11·5 years (males) and 23 years (females), whereas for rural York, they are markedly longer: 15 years (males) and 30 years (females).

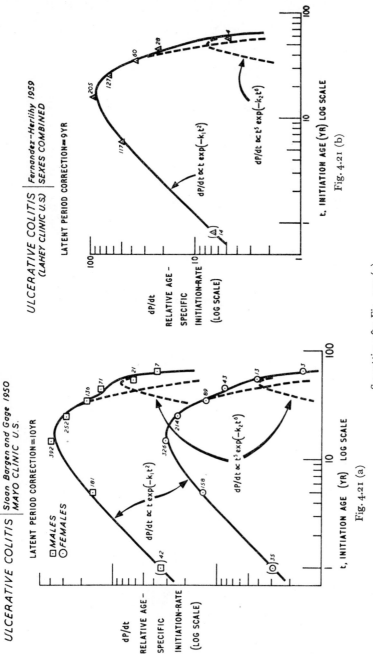

ULCERATIVE COLITIS | Sloan Bargen and Gage 1950
MAYO CLINIC U.S.

LATENT PERIOD CORRECTION = 10YR

□ MALES
○ FEMALES

dP/dt ∝ t exp(−k₁t²)

dP/dt ∝ t⁵ exp(−k₂t⁹)

dP/dt
RELATIVE AGE –
SPECIFIC
INITIATION-RATE
(LOG SCALE)

t, INITIATION AGE (YR) LOG SCALE

Fig. 4·21 (a)

ULCERATIVE COLITIS | Fernandez–Herlihy 1959
(LAHEY CLINIC U.S.) SEXES COMBINED

LATENT PERIOD CORRECTION = 9YR

dP/dt ∝ t exp(−k₁t²)

dP/dt ∝ t⁵ exp(−k₂t⁹)

dP/dt
RELATIVE AGE –
SPECIFIC
INITIATION-RATE
(LOG SCALE)

t, INITIATION AGE (YR) LOG SCALE

Fig. 4·21 (b)

See caption after Fig. 4·21 (g)

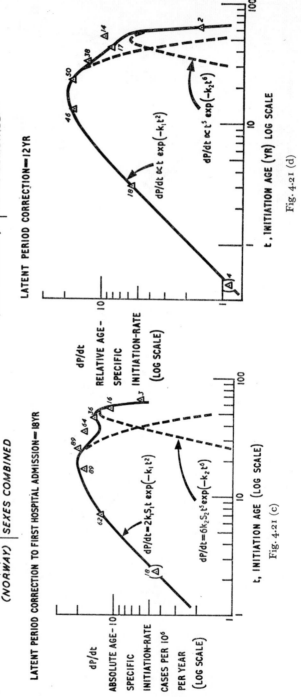

ULCERATIVE COLITIS | Wigley and Maclaurin 1962
(NEW ZEALAND) | SEXES COMBINED

LATENT PERIOD CORRECTION=12YR

$dP/dt \propto t \exp(-k_1 t^2)$

$dP/dt \propto t^5 \exp(-k_2 t^6)$

t, INITIATION AGE (YR) LOG SCALE

Fig. 4·21 (d)

dP/dt

RELATIVE AGE- SPECIFIC INITIATION-RATE (LOG SCALE)

See caption after Fig. 4·21 (g)

ULCERATIVE COLITIS | Ustvedt 1958
(NORWAY) | SEXES COMBINED

LATENT PERIOD CORRECTION TO FIRST HOSPITAL ADMISSION=18YR

dP/dt

ABSOLUTE AGE- SPECIFIC INITIATION-RATE CASES PER 10^6 PER YEAR (LOG SCALE)

$dP/dt = 2k_1S_1 t \exp(-k_1 t^2)$

$dP/dt = 6k_2S_2 t^5 \exp(-k_2 t^6)$

t, INITIATION AGE (LOG SCALE)

Fig. 4·21 (c)

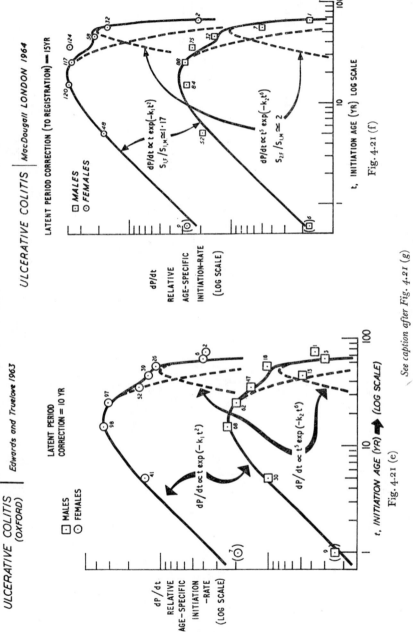

ULCERATIVE COLITIS (OXFORD) | Edwards and Truelove 1963

ULCERATIVE COLITIS | MacDougall LONDON 1964

See caption after Fig. 4·21 (g)

Fig. 4·21 (e)

Fig. 4·21 (f)

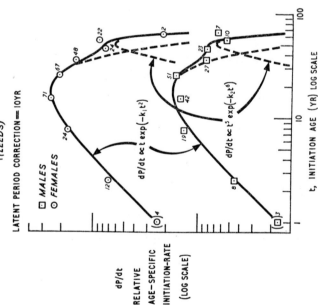

Fig. 4·21 Seven large clinical series of ulcerative colitis from: (a) the Mayo Clinic, U.S. (Sloan *et al.* 1950); (b) Lahey Clinic, U.S. (Fernandez-Herlihy 1959); (c) Norway (Ustvedt 1958); (d) New Zealand (Wigley and Maclaurin 1962); and England – (e) Oxford (Edwards and Truelove 1963); (f) London (MacDougall 1964); and (g) Leeds (de Dombal 1967a). All the data are fitted to the same two stochastic equations, with the same value of k_1 ($1·54 \times 10^{-3}$ yr^{-2}) and k_2 ($5·3 \times 10^{-11}$ yr^{-6}). Proportions of early to late onset cases, (genotypes 1 and 2), and sex-ratios, differ from series to series reflecting differences in the geographical distribution of the predisposing genes. Where latent period corrections are comparable (to first onset) these range from 9 years (Lahey Clinic, U.S. series) to 12 years (New Zealand). Uniformity in the age patterns k on geography and time – is seen with Huntington's chorea (Burch 1968a); and a classical 'autoimmune' disease, chronic discoid lupus erythematosus (Burch and Rowell 1968).

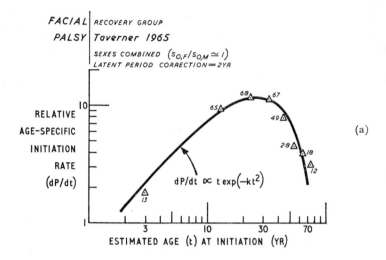

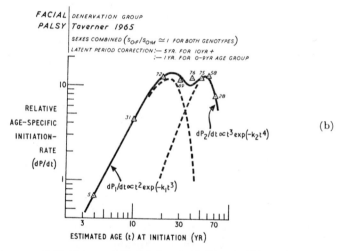

Fig. 4.22 a and b. Taverner's (1965) data for facial palsy. Illustrating a disease in which three distinctive groups are involved. The recovery group can be distinguished clinically from the two denervation groups. For the recovery group: $r = 2$, and $k \simeq 6 \cdot 6 \times 10^{-4}$ yr^{-2}; for the denervation group with a modal initiation age of 23 years: $r = 3$, and $k_1 \simeq 5 \cdot 5 \times 10^{-5}$ yr^{-3}; and for the second denervation group: $r = 4$, and $k_2 \simeq 8 \cdot 2 \times 10^{-8}$ yr^{-4}. No significant sex differences are seen in any of the parameters including the latent period.

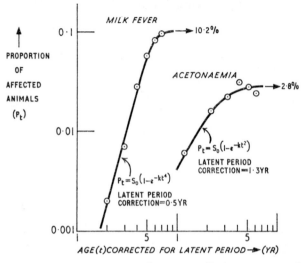

DISEASES IN THE BRITISH DAIRY HERD
DATA FROM: *DISEASE WASTAGE AND HUSBANDRY 1957-58*
BULLETIN OF MINISTRY OF AGRICULTURE (1960)

Fig. 4.23 To illustrate that diseases manifesting autoaggressive statistics are not confined to man. I am indebted to my colleague Mr K. G. Towers for drawing my attention to these veterinary statistics (Ministry of Agriculture 1960).

CLASSES OF DISEASE: CORRESPONDENCE BETWEEN STATISTICS, ANATOMY, AND CLINICAL EVIDENCE

From the examples given it will be seen that the age-patterns of many diseases can be divided into two broad classes: (i) those in which the *average latent period* (λ) *in a given environment is of equal duration in the two sexes*; and (ii) those where the *average latent period in females* (λ_F) *is twice as long as in males* (λ_M). In this latter circumstance (which can be regarded as a special form of genetic heterogeneity, that is, sex-differentiation) I have concluded that the endogenous defence against the proliferating forbidden-clone(s) is twice as efficient in females as in similarly-predisposed males (Burch 1963c). This conclusion is well supported by clinical evidence: in systemic lupus erythematosus, prognosis is markedly better for women than men (Kellum and Haserick 1964) although many more females are predisposed to the disease (Burch and Rowell

1965a). Hale and Scowen (1967) find that in myasthenia gravis with thymic tumours, the 5-year survival is 48 per cent for males and 70 per cent for females; the 10-year survival is 24 per cent (males) and 48 per cent (females). In Dupuytren's contracture, where again $\lambda_F = 2\lambda_M$, Hueston (1963) found that 27·6 per cent of men over 60 with the disorder showed flexion deformity, whereas only 14·3 per cent of women in this age group were thus afflicted. On the other hand, in ulcerative colitis, where $\lambda_F = \lambda_M$, de Dombal (1967a) finds no significant sex-differences in the frequency of acute attacks. In Huntington's chorea $\lambda_F = \lambda_M$, and in a U.S. series of patients, Chandler *et al.* (1960) found that the mean interval between the onset of chorea and death was 15·8 years for males and 15·9 years for females; the corresponding intervals found by Panse (1942) in Germany were 13·9 and 13·0 years, respectively. Once again, the agreement between theory and clinical studies powerfully supports the validity of the detailed mathematical analysis of age patterns, including the estimation of latent periods, and the interpretation of their biological significance.

So far as we have been able to judge, latent periods are the same in the two sexes whenever the immediate target tissue of the primary autoaggressive attack lies normally behind a blood-tissue barrier. Central and peripheral nervous systems, articular cartilage, and bone, are classical examples of such tissues. The initial direct attack on cells in such tissues must obviously be carried out by humoral as opposed to cellular agents (but *not* by immunoglobulin autoantibodies – see Chapter 7). When tissues are normally freely infiltrated by small lymphocytes (e.g. synovium and the endothelial lining of arteries) the latent period in autoaggressive diseases of such tissues is twice as long in females as in males.

The histopathological evidence for diseases in which $\lambda_F = 2\lambda_M$, is consistent with the view that the primary 'autoantibodies' are cellular (Burch 1963c; Burch and Rowell 1965a); they probably constitute repeating units of the plasma membrane of one class of small lymphocyte. When the target tissue of the autoaggressive attack lies behind a blood-tissue barrier, the serological evidence suggests that the primary autoantibody usually migrates on electrophoresis with the α_2-globulin fraction; from immunoelectrophoresis of serum proteins it seems likely that an α_2-macroglobulin fraction is often implicated (Burch and Burwell 1965; Burch and Rowell 1965b; Burch 1968a).

RECAPITULATION

A brief summary of the more important provisional conclusions that can be drawn from the mathematical analysis of the age-patterns of disease may be appropriate at this juncture.

Ageing consists, in the main, of a very large number of specific autoaggressive disorders. (Most forms of malignant cancer are excluded from this generalisation.) The whole, or nearly the whole population appears to be at risk with respect to some autoaggressive disorders, whereas others are confined to specific sub-populations ranging in size from a large to a very small fraction of the general population. Genetic factors – monogenic or polygenic – distinguish predisposed individuals from the non-predisposed; sex-linked factors are commonly, but not invariably found. All autoaggressive disorders are initiated by random events, which have some remarkable properties. Their number is usually small, and they may occur in 1, up to at least 5 cells; perhaps as many as 12 events can occur in a single cell. A specific event, for a specific disease, occurs at the same average rate, in similarly-predisposed individuals, from birth, or even before birth, to the end of the life-span; rates are not perceptibly affected by ordinary environments. The average rate of a given initiating event in XX females is either the same as, or double that, in similarly-predisposed XY males. At the end of the initiation-phase, when the full complement of random initiating events has occurred, an interval or latent period elapses before symptoms or signs of the disease emerge. This interval can be affected by various ordinary environmental factors, but in a given environment, its average duration in females is either equal to, or double that in males.

Study of age-patterns is essential to the full genetic analysis of age-dependent disease, and a comprehensive catalogue is much to be desired, especially for genetic counselling. Inter-

pretation of sex- and age-distributions is necessary to the understanding of the causes of disease and ageing. Am I really
justified, however, in postulating a pathogenic role for those
seemingly inexorable, and therefore immensely unpopular
somatic mutations? I devote the next chapter to this question.

5. ARE THE INITIATING EVENTS RANDOM SOMATIC MUTATIONS?

'The general problem of mathematical statistics is that of stochastic models: given a distribution – what is the chance mechanism that generated it?'

Jerzy Neyman, 1967

Suppose we find ourselves blessed with accurate and abundant age-statistics for a genetically-based disease. Suppose the statistics come from several well-defined and well-separated populations, at different secular times. Let us further imagine all these impeccable sets of data to be consistent with one of the models described in the previous chapter. That is to say, the same n and/or r values are obtained from each set of data, and the k values do not differ significantly, one from another. (The value of S, which depends on gene frequencies, can be expected to differ from population to population; the value of λ can also differ as the result of various environmental factors.) Does it then follow that the pathogenesis of the disease has to be explained in terms of the relevant stochastic model of the last chapter? Or is there a better solution avoiding those detested somatic mutations?

I have to concede there is no *logical necessity* for the specific interpretation given, or indeed, for any other scientific interpretation of quantitative empirical evidence. We could argue that the age-patterns of disease reflect acts of God – or more plausibly, acts of the devil. (The argument is difficult to refute.) Alternatively, we might propose that each individual is equipped with many 'biological clocks' which 'time' the onset of the various idiopathic diseases by some sequential, clock-like mechanism. We would then be obliged to demonstrate the biological nature and functioning of each 'clock'. Also, we would have to admit that by a fantastic set of coincidences, the biological clock-settings for a specific disease, in many geographically – and temporally – separated populations, are always distributed to agree with the same version of the general stochastic equation [4.7]. This is a great weakness of the 'clock' argument. It is simply not credible that sequential, *deterministic* biological clocks, are distributed among individuals, in many different populations, so that they always 'go off' according to the general *stochastic* equation [4.7]. Moreover, monozygotic twins seldom succumb to specific autoaggressive disorders at the same age.

Such considerations make it very difficult, or even impossible, to devise any realistic non-stochastic interpretation of those age-patterns that conform to: $P_t = S(1-e^{-kt})^n$, or the differential form of this equation. When, as with clinical inflammatory polyarthritis (Burch 1966c, 1968b), the severity of the disease is related to the value of n, I am unaware of any plausible alternative to the view that n describes the number of forbidden-clones, where each arises from one stem cell, in each of n independent sets of stem cells. However, when age-patterns follow Weibull statistics (equations [4.4] and [4.5]) the biological interpretation is not immediately obvious, and several possibilities have to be considered. These equations would be obeyed if, for example, a single random event (mutation) in each of r contiguous (touching) cells had to occur to initiate the disease process (Fisher and Hollman 1951). Fisher (1958) has described another possibility. Suppose r is found to be 4. This could be interpreted in terms of the following sequence: (i) an initial spontaneous somatic mutation in any one of L cells; (ii) the growth of a clone from the mutant cell such that, after the first few divisions, the number of cells in the clone increases with the square of time, and then finally; (iii) to initiate the disease, a further spontaneous somatic mutation is needed in any one of the (singly) mutant clonal cells.

We cannot distinguish between these and similar models on mathematical grounds alone, and we have to appeal to cytological, immunological, and biochemical considerations, to decide between the alternatives. Where autoaggressive disease is concerned, Fisher's (1958) model is an unpromising candidate because it is unlikely that stage (ii) would be independent of environmental factors such as diet and infections. So far as I can see from the available evidence, the age-pattern of initiation is virtually invariant with respect to such factors. With accurate statistics, data can be fitted to equation [4.4], (or better, its differentiated form) with *integral* values of r : 2, 3, 4, etc., and this would be rather unlikely if clonal growth (stage (ii)) were a common occurrence. Fisher and Hollman's 'contiguous cell' model is also suspect in the autoaggressive context, because, if such an anatomical relationship were essential at the stem cell level, it would probably have to be maintained throughout the proliferating clone. Furthermore, although it is often found that when $r \geqslant 2$, the value of k in females is twice the value of k in males, I have not yet found an instance of k being four times, or eight times . . . etc., higher. If the mutation of an X-linked gene in each of r contiguous cells is ever involved, then rates in females would be 2^r times higher than in males. The failure, so far, to observe such rate differences between the sexes suggests that the 'r contiguous cell' model is seldom (if ever) relevant.

In the context of acute leukaemia in childhood (see Chapter 11) the findings from patients with Down's syndrome (mongolism) and from those without, provide cogent reasons for adopting the model of 'r mutations in one cell'. However, the definitive solution to the interpretation of 'r' in most other age-patterns will have to await direct immunological and/or biochemical analyses of specific proteins, synthesised by normal and mutant cells. Suffice it to say that, the existing evidence favours the simplest view – that the value of r is equal to the number of mutations required in a single stem cell to initiate the disease process.

I conclude therefore that the general equations [4.6] and [4.7] are best interpreted in terms of the following simple biological model: (i) spontaneous somatic gene mutations are needed to initiate the disease; (ii) from birth to death, gene instability follows a law of the same form as the law of radioactive decay; (iii) multiple somatic mutations may occur in independent cells (to give Yule statistics), but also in any one cell, out of a population of cells (to give Weibull statistics). As yet, no biologically realistic alternative to the broad stochastic interpretation described in Chapter 4 is in sight. However, when in the context of autoaggressive disease r is greater than 2, we have to bear in mind the possibility (and it is little more than a possibility) that one or more intermediate stages of clonal growth might occur, sandwiched in between random events. Clearly, we have to make predictions from our model, and we have to test their consequences against experiment, observation, and general scientific principles. In the next two chapters, I show that this model leads to some exceptionally precise predictions.

Although the sceptic may concede that the initiating events occur randomly, does it necessarily follow that they are a form of gene mutation? Again, I cannot claim logical necessity. But is it even remotely plausible to contend that infective, or traumatic, or dietary, or allergic, or psychic stress episodes could occur randomly, *and* at an average rate that is constant from birth to death, *and* from country to country, *and* at different times? *and* could their average rate of occurrence in women be either the same as that in men, or twice as high? *and* could they consistently conform either to Yule, or to Weibull statistics or to a combination of the two? To each of these several questions we are forced to give an emphatic NO! It would be ludicrous to attribute such properties to extrinsic factors of the kind mentioned above.

In contrast, we encounter no difficulty when the initiating events are regarded as somatic mutations. Furthermore, deep significance must attach to the finding that rates are constant throughout postnatal life – indicating that the number (L) of cells at risk is constant – and that rates in XX females can be double those in XY males – suggesting that both homologous X-linked genes can be at risk in females. (In only one obvious respect do XX females differ from XY males in the quantitative ratio of 2 to 1.) I shall return to these points in the next chapter, and I shall describe further evidence supporting the mutation theory of the initiating events in Chapter 11.

SOMATIC GENE MUTATION-RATES

Age-patterns often enable us to define k quite accurately, but they do not yield the value of L, the number of cells at risk, or the rate of gene mutation, m. But suppose that in a given disease $k = Lm_1 . m_2 \ldots m_r$ (which we can write as Lm^r, where m is an effective mean rate for each of the r genes), then if we can choose a reasonable upper limit to L, this will define a lower limit for m. Oppositely, we can select a lower limit to L, to define an upper limit for m in a given disease. (In general, we may expect m to differ markedly from locus to locus, because this is found in germ cells, where mutation rates can often be ascertained more directly.)

The total number of myeloid stem cells in adult bone marrow has been estimated (Burch 1965) to be of the order of 10^{10}, and hence it is exceedingly unlikely that the number of cells at risk in any tissue-specific autoaggressive disease will be greater than – or even as great as – 10^{10}. Considering coronary artery disease in adults, where the value of r is 6 (Fig. 4.10), the value of L is not very critical in calculating the mean value m. (An error of six orders of magnitude in L will result in an error of one order of magnitude in m.) We find $k = Lm^r = 3 \cdot 2 \times 10^{-12}$ yr^{-6}, and hence, putting $L = 10^{10}$ as an upper limit, we obtain $m \geqslant 2 \cdot 5 \times 10^{-4}$ per year.

We are now confronted with the difficult task of setting a lower limit to L so that we can find an upper limit for m in an appropriate disease. From investigations of acute radiation death in mice (Upton *et al.* 1956), I have concluded that the value of L for a critical set of growth-control stem cells might be ~ 20 (see Chapter 10).

If we now consider a specific autoaggressive condition such as dental caries in first permanent molars, where the k value is relatively high, we find $k(= Lm) \simeq 0 \cdot 3$ per year (that is, $0 \cdot 3$ yr^{-1}). Hence, putting $L = 20$ as a lower limit, we obtain $m < 1 \cdot 5 \times 10^{-2}$ yr^{-1}. Because m may sometimes be greater than $2 \cdot 5 \times 10^{-4}$ yr^{-1}, values in the region of 10^{-3} yr^{-1} may not be altogether unrepresentative, although wide differences from one gene to another should be anticipated.

This rate is very high when compared with previously estimated mutation frequencies for germ cells in man. In the present units (rate per *year* and not per generation) typical germ cell mutation frequencies are $\sim 10^{-6}$ per gene, per gamete, per year, although values up to 2×10^{-4} yr^{-1} have been claimed (see Burch 1965).

Comparison with certain spontaneous mutation-rates in bacteria, is, however, most intriguing. Novick and Szilard (1950) determined the rate of mutation to resistance to bacteriophage T5 in a strain (B/1) of *E. coli*. They were able to vary the generation time of bacteria in their chemostat over the range 2 to 12 hours. Defining the mutation-rate per generation as p, and the generation time as τ, they found p/τ to be constant, and equal to $1 \cdot 25 \times 10^{-8}$ hr^{-1} at $37°C$, or $1 \cdot 1 \times 10^{-4}$ yr^{-1}. It was about half this value at $25°C$. They commented: 'If mutants arose for instance, as the result of some error in the process of gene duplication, then one would hardly expect the probability of a mutation occurring per cell division to be inversely proportionate to the rate of growth. If the process of mutation could be considered as a monomolecular reaction – as had been once suggested by Delbrück and Timoféeff-Ressovsky – then, of course, the rate of mutation per unit time should be constant.'

This observed rate of a particular spontaneous mutation in bacteria is about an order of magnitude less than the very approximate value for certain genes in human somatic cells mentioned above. However, in the broad context of mutation-rates, an order of magnitude is neither here nor there, and the detailed kinetics of the bacterial events, and the general properties of the mammalian events, are both consistent with the view that these mutations involve a unimolecular reaction. It is difficult to attribute these random changes in gene expression to errors in DNA replication. I pursue this mutational problem in Chapter 7.

6. IMPLICATIONS OF THE SEX- AND AGE-PATTERNS OF DISEASE FOR NORMAL GROWTH-CONTROL

'The object of reasoning is to find out, from the consideration of what we already know, something else which we do not know. Consequently, reasoning is good if it be such as to give a true conclusion from true premises, and not otherwise.'

C. S. Peirce

We have become so familiar with the notion of biological variability that the remarkable fit of the age-distributions of so many diseases to a very simple biological model is unexpected. Sometimes we find that a disease such as psoriasis (Burch and Rowell 1965b) or ulcerative colitis (Fig. 4.21), is not genetically homogeneous, and that two groups can be distinguished by age-pattern analysis, and confirmed by detailed clinical and/or genetic studies. Occasionally, as with facial (Bell's) palsy, three distinctive groups can be delineated (see Figs 4.22a and b). Given sufficiently refined diagnostic criteria, it seems likely that a genuinely specific disease within this general class is always confined to a single genetically-distinctive group of people. Indeed, by ordinary current diagnostic criteria, many diseases appear to be of this category. This is also surprising. Instead of finding a variable, genetically-determined *gradation* of susceptibility to age-dependent diseases, *with everyone more or less at risk*, we encounter qualitative distinctions: either we are predisposed, or we are not. Of course, given the predisposition, the severity of the disease can vary widely from time to time within the same patient, and it can also show marked differences from one patient to another. But you will never get psoriasis, in any form, unless you have a specific genetic predisposition to that skin disorder.

GENE ACTION IN AUTOAGGRESSIVE DISEASE

Consider why a specific gene, or combination of genes, is needed to predispose to a particular, and narrowly-defined autoaggressive disease, and why the number of initiating somatic mutations is unique.

Immune relationships between classical antigen and antibody are characterised by their great specificity, and they are believed to depend on a complementary 'fit' of the lock and key, or male and female type, between the combining site on the antibody, and the antigenic determinant. The *complementary steric relationship* between these two structures is the basis of the classical antibody-antigen reaction. If we change the shape of the antibody binding-site, affinity for the original antigen is lost; and equally, if we change the shape of the antigenic determinant, combination with the original antibody is prevented.

From transplantation and other studies, especially those of blood groups, it is well known that cells are characterised immunologically by multiple antigenic determinants. Certain histocompatibility antigens are shared by many tissues, whereas other antigens are confined to specific tissues: they are *tissue specific antigens*. We use our omnibus term *tissue coding factor* (TCF), to describe all the 'antigenic' (recognition) features of the plasma membrane of a cell (Burch and Burwell 1965). 'Mutant' molecules – in other words, primary (non-immunoglobulin) autoantibodies – attack a particular target tissue, or tissues to produce autoaggressive disease. One TCF will be 'hit' by a complementary autoantibody in say, autoimmune thyroiditis, but in autoimmune haemolytic anaemia, a different TCF will be attacked by its own complementary autoantibody . . . and so on. Each specific autoaggressive disease is associated with one or more autoantibodies that are specific to that disease, and to the affected target tissue(s).

THREE POSSIBILITIES

When we consider the part played by predisposing genes in autoaggressive disease, three obvious possibilities arise (Burch 1963c). (1) The predisposing genes code in mesenchymal (M) cells for polypeptide chains forming a part, or the whole, of the molecule that, at the end of the initiation phase, becomes the primary autoantibody. (2) They code in target (T) cells for some, or all, of the antigenic determinants of the tissue coding factor (TCF). (3) They perform both (1) and (2) – that is, they help to determine the structure both of the future autoantibody, and of the TCFs synthesised by target (T) cells.

Consider (1). Suppose that genes a, b, and c predispose to a particular autoaggressive disease, and suppose the disease is initiated by somatic mutation, in a mesenchymal stem cell, of genes p, q, and r to their allelic forms, p_m, q_m, and r_m, respectively. If p, q, and r can mutate in somatic cells, they should also mutate in germ cells. It follows that individuals with the a, b, and c predisposing genes should be found in whom, say, the mutant gene p_m has also been inherited; this mutant gene will be transmitted to all somatic cells – apart from further somatic mutation, which we can ignore. Individuals with this particular predisposition, a, b, c, and p_m, should require only 2 somatic mutations (of the q and r genes), to initiate the autoaggressive disease. Broadening the argument, if an autoaggressive disease is initiated by, say, 6 somatic mutations in one genotype, then five other genotypes should be present in the population requiring 5, 4, 3, 2, and 1 initiating somatic mutations, respectively.

As we have seen, the evidence flatly contradicts this prediction. Hence the premises, and/or the argument must be false. The closest approach to this prediction I have met so far is provided by Bell's palsy, where three distinctive genotypes are found, requiring 2, 3, and 4 initiating somatic mutations, respectively (Figs 4.22 a and b). This, however, is an exceptional example, and even here, no genotype is found requiring only one somatic mutation.

To rescue the simple model (1), we could postulate that genotypes containing the mutant genes p_m, and/or q_m, and/or r_m, are lethal. However, the evidence reveals numerous genes of the p, q, r type, and their rate of mutation, at least in somatic cells, is very high (see previous chapter). It is very unlikely, therefore, that any genotype could exist without genes of the form p_m, etc., being present. Model (1), in original or modified forms, is therefore highly unpropitious – to say the least.

Consider hypothesis (2). If predisposing genes a, b, and c code for the TCF, and if the 'autoantibody genes' in M cells are entirely independent, then in general we would expect to find some individuals in the population with M cells requiring only 1 mutation, others requiring 2, 3 . . . etc., mutations to initiate the disease. As we have just seen in connection with model (1) this expectation is not realised. Model (2) is therefore falsified in the same kind of way as model (1).

That leaves us with model (3): predisposing genes code for recognition polypeptide chains both in M and in T cells. This differs fundamentally from (1) and (2) because in (3), when germ cell mutations produce individuals with allele p_m – as well as genes a, b, and c – then p_m will contribute to the structure of proteins *both* in M *and* in T cells. Although only 2 subsequent somatic mutations (to q_m and r_m) are required in an M cell of an 'a, b, c, p_m' individual to produce an 'auto-antibody' identical in structure with the usual autoantibody, the autoaggressive disease does not develop. This is because the allele p_m, instead of p, codes for a polypeptide chain of the TCF to produce a different structure. Whereas the 'a, b, c, p' TCF is attacked autoaggressively by the complementary 'a, b, c, p_m, q_m, r_m' M-cell protein, the sterically different 'a, b, c, p_m' TCF, is not susceptible. In this way model (3) explains how an autoaggressive disease, affecting a specific tissue, with a specific TCF, can be confined to a single genetically-predisposed group, and why the number of somatic mutations needed to produce the autoantibody, and therefore to initiate the disease, is unique. Individuals outside the predisposed group have, by definition, TCFs that are sterically-dissimilar from those which are vulnerable to clinically-detectable disease.

Many of the above considerations will have applications to the equally challenging problem of carcinogenesis.

In view of the great variety in the numbers of somatic mutations needed to initiate autoaggressive disorders (from 1 to at least 18), and considering that genetic predisposition may be monogenic (dominant or recessive), or polygenic (up to at least 5 loci), the rules governing autoaggressive interactions are evidently very complicated. These rules should be derivable from protein chemistry (and hence, ultimately, from the laws of quantum mechanics) but because we do not yet understand the mechanism of even the simplest enzyme-substrate reaction, it will be some time before we can hope to command a working knowledge of the terrifyingly complex interaction between primary autoantibody and TCF.

IMPLICATIONS OF MODEL (3)

Suppose that genes a, b, c, d, e, f, and g, code in T cells for the multiple polypeptide chains of the TCF, and in mutant or non-mutant form, for the polypeptide chains in M cell auto-antibodies. (The generally small *proportion* of T cells with 'mutant TCFs' does not concern us in this context.) Suppose the fraction S of the population predisposed to the disease is less than unity. Then according to model (3), at least one of the a to g genes, with alleles in homozygous or heterozygous arrangement, will feature in the predisposing genotype. It follows that, in some circumstances the predisposing allele or alleles might themselves mutate in M cells to initiate the forbidden-clone. This possibility is indeed supported by the evidence for autoaggressive disease. To take a simple example, predisposition to systemic lupus erythematosus (where the ratio, S_F/S_M, of predisposed females to males in the United States is about 4·5) probably involves *three* dominant effect X-linked genes (as well as autosomal factors) and initiation occurs through the independent somatic mutation of *three* X-linked genes in M cells (Burch and Rowell 1965a). Either we have struck a remarkable coincidence, or the predisposing X-linked genes undergo mutation in lymphoid stem cells to initiate the disease. Other parallels between the predisposing genotype and the initiating events have been described elsewhere (Burch 1964c; Burch and Rowell 1965b).

From the foregoing arguments we therefore conclude that genes predisposing to an autoaggressive disease perform a dual function: *they direct the synthesis of polypeptide chains both in M (mesenchymal) cells and in target (T) cells.* Consequently, there should be an identity relation between parts (at least) of normal M cell proteins, and parts (at least) of their normal target tissue TCFs. Moreover, this identity relation should extend to every mesenchyme-TCF system that can be involved in autoaggressive ('autoimmune') disease. An exclusive relation of this kind, applying to so many different tissues, must surely have profound biological significance.

GENETIC, MOLECULAR, AND PHYSICO-CHEMICAL BASIS OF GROWTH-CONTROL

We already know (see Jehle 1963) that London/van der Waal's charge-fluctuation forces produce a specific attraction between *identical* complex molecules. (The phenomena of dimer and polymer formation provide notorious complications when determining the molecular weights of proteins.) For obvious reasons, and very appropriately for us, these highly specific, but rather weak and short-range forces of attraction, are called *self-recognition* forces.

At last, we have arrived at a solution to what is, perhaps, the major enigma in Burwell's (1963) growth theory – or, indeed, of any theory of growth-control by a central system: How do growth-control effectors recognise the correct target tissue, and how do target tissue affectors recognise their own control element? In Chapter 2, I called the complex molecules making up mesenchymal (M) mitogenic effectors *mitotic control proteins* (MCPs), and these can be humoral – perhaps α_2-macro-globulins synthesised by cells of the basophil-mast cell series – or cellular – one class of small lymphocyte. A specific MCP homes onto, and interacts with, its cognate TCF on the target cell plasma membrane, because both the MCP and the TCF are made up of a number of identical polypeptide chains, and because London *self-recognition* forces operate between identical complex components. Similarly, humoral afferent TCFs locate, and interact with, their cognate receptor cells in the M system bearing MCPs on their plasma membrane, through the same kind of self-recognition interaction mechanism. (Probably – see Chapter 11 – afferent TCFs are first 'processed,' through the removal of lipids by enzymes in macrophagic cells, before being presented to receptor M cells to regulate the release of effectors (Ballantyne and Burwell 1965).) Whether the inter-molecular MCP–TCF interaction occurs directly through 'contact' between identical sections of the folded MCP and TCF polypeptide chains, or through contact between prosthetic groups such as lipids and/or carbohydrates attached to the protein is, of course, unresolved by the present argument. My reasoning merely defines the *underlying* genetic and molecular basis of mutual MCP–TCF recognition.

Because the number of distinctive tissues in mammals is astronomical, the economy of using one set of genes to determine the steric specificity of MCPs *and* TCFs is obvious. The two way recognition problem in the negative-feedback growth-control loop, is solved in the simplest possible way. Evolution may safely be credited with such economical tendencies.

CAN THERE BE AN ALTERNATIVE GENETIC BASIS FOR GROWTH-CONTROL?

Having arrived at one solution to the genetic and molecular basis of central growth-control, we must now consider whether any alternative basis is possible. Although plausible, the above arguments are not decisive. The age-patterns, and the familial evidence for many diseases, show that they are *largely* confined to one or a few distinctive genotypes. But in the absence of sophisticated immunological and/or biochemical tests of the specificity of MCPs, TCFs and autoantibodies we cannot, as yet, be absolutely certain that our induction is valid, and that every victim has a specific inheritance. Neither can we be sure that model (3) excludes all other alternatives.

I now proceed to a new argument (Burch 1966c), which leads to the same conclusion, and which, so far as I can see, is decisive. An alternative genetic basis for mutual MCP–TCF recognition would, by definition, have to use one set of genes to code for MCPs, and a non-identical set to code for TCFs. Now the total amount of DNA in the nucleus of the mammalian cell (about 6×10^{-12} g) will specify about 6×10^6 genes, if each gene codes for a polypeptide chain of average molecular weight 20 000 daltons (Burch and Burwell 1965; Comings 1967). Most of these genes are likely to be involved in MCP–TCF coding – a point of the utmost important which, hitherto, has been largely if not completely overlooked. For simplicity, suppose 10^6 genes are used, in the appropriate combinations, to code for a very much larger number ($?10^8$) of MCPs; and that another, and entirely different 10^6 genes are used, also in the appropriate combinations, for TCF coding. In view of the extremely exacting demands on the precision of recognition, point mutation of an 'MCP gene' in the germ cell would often disrupt MCP–TCF recognition, and analogous point mutation of a 'TCF gene' would have the same disastrous effect. In man, typical germ cell mutation-rates are of the order of 10^{-5} per gene, per gamete, per generation. Hence, if our complete MCP–TCF system were perfectly matched for mutual recognition in generation 1, we might expect ∼40 errors in the next generation, resulting in the collapse of 40 growth-control elements, to be followed by the collapse of a further 40 in the next generation . . . etc., to extinction. This failure-rate is clearly exorbitant because the loss of even one element might occasionally be fatal. A species relying on one set of genes for MCP coding, and a different set for TCF coding, could never survive.

Furthermore, we must not forget that evolutionary change towards complexity has been contingent upon the admission of certain point mutations, and the addition of genetic 'information', to the germ cell lines. Hence, the use of a common set of genes for MCP–TCF coding is a prerequisite for the evolution of complex multi-tissue organisms. Point mutations in growth-control genes will be acceptable to their inheritors, provided the resulting configuration and properties of both MCPs and TCFs, cellular and humoral, are compatible with their overall function.

This second argument for the identity of MCP and TCF mutual 'recognition genes' rests on four empirical premises, and it is entirely independent of the first, which derives in part from inductions from the evidence for autoaggressive diseases. The four premises are: (i) organisms such as man consist of a very large number of distinctive tissues; (ii) beyond a certain stage of embryogenesis, the symmetrical mitosis of target cells during normal growth is controlled by a central system; (iii) one tissue is distinguished from another by tissue coding factors (TCFs), the steric specificity of which is related to gene specificity; and (iv) genes mutate.

I have contended – not without trepidation – that a fundamentally different scheme could not have evolved; no other genetic basis for the central control and co-ordination of growth in complex multi-tissue organisms is feasible. This contention has a quality of absoluteness which is likely to be deeply disturbing to some people who, like myself, have been fed a diet of logical positivism, philosophical analysis,

Heisenberg's famous Uncertainty Principle, and the principles of verification and falsification – not to mention the writings of Karl Popper. We have been taught that empirical laws – as opposed to the tautologies of pure mathematics and formal logic – can never be known to be absolutely true: consistency between our scientific theory and the best observations made to date, is the most we can expect, or even hope for. A new and more accurate measurement made tomorrow might always reveal unsuspected defects in our most carefully thought-out theory.

A loophole would be attractive, and one escape from the uncomfortable absolute position concerning the genetic and molecular basis of growth-control might still be open: the form of growth that involves symmetrical mitosis of cells might not be centrally controlled after all. Instead, each specific tissue might contain its own control: premise (ii) might be false. However, the experimental evidence reviewed below blocks even this escape route.

IS NORMAL GROWTH CENTRALLY CONTROLLED?

Investigations of the abscopal effects of ionising radiation on the growth of various organs show that damage outside the organ is far more important than radiation injury to the organ itself. For example, Conard (1964) has found that the growth of a tibia in a rat shows a much greater decrement when the bone is shielded from radiation and the remainder of the body is irradiated, than when the body is shielded and the tibia is irradiated. Compensatory growth is similarly revealing. It is well known that if one kidney is removed from a healthy animal, the remaining kidney roughly doubles its size. Wachtel and Cole (1965) removed one kidney from a young growing rat and exteriorised the other one. To one group of animals treated in this way, they delivered a large dose (1000 rad) of X-rays to the exteriorised kidney, while shielding the rest of the animal's body. They found that whole-body growth was unaffected, and only a small decrement in compensatory growth occurred in the heavily-irradiated kidney. However, another group of uninephrectomised young rats received a smaller dose (500 rad) of X-rays to the 'whole' body, while the exteriorised kidney was shielded; in this experiment there was a retardation of whole-body growth, and a marked reduction in compensatory growth of the remaining kidney. So, in the experiments of Conard (1964), and of Wachtel and Cole (1965), the abscopal, or indirect effect of damaging radiation on the growth of an organ, is far more pronounced than the direct effect.

The favoured organ in studies of regenerative growth in mammals is the liver of the rat; when a part of this organ (typically two of the three lobes) is removed from a young animal, the remaining part of the liver grows, and within a month, the total size of the regenerated liver approximates to the size of the normal organ. Some ingenious experiments of Leong *et al.* (1964), and Virolainen (1964), show that the stimulus to regenerative growth is blood-borne. These authors first transplanted small specimens of the liver of an animal to subcutaneous sites within the same animal: these are 'heterotopic partial autografts'. Following recovery from this operation, partial hepatectomy was performed, and it was found that the rate of mitosis in the autografts increased in the same way, and in the same time relation, as those in the remaining liver lobe. Hence, some systemic factor affected liver tissue simultaneously, regardless of its anatomical location. Attempts to demonstrate a humoral mitogenic agent have met with variable success – see a review by Bucher (1967) – although in recent cross-circulation experiments, Moolten and Bucher (1967) have shown that a humoral factor from a partially-hepatectomised rat stimulates mitosis in the hepatocytes of a normal rat. Difficulties in detecting humoral mitogenic factors are not surprising, because in theory, the serum of an animal contains both mitogenic agents (humoral MCPs) and factors indirectly inhibiting symmetrical mitosis (affector humoral TCFs inhibiting the release of MCPs). Regeneration of the ductular cells of liver may in any case require cellular MCPs (small lymphocytes), because the peak mitotic-rate in these cells following partial hepatectomy occurs later than in the parenchymal cells. In heterotopic (subcutaneous) autografts, the ductular cells, unlike parenchymal cells, do not respond to the mitotic stimulus provided by partial hepatectomy.

The quantitative description of liver regeneration in relation to time after partial hepatectomy is of considerable theoretical interest. If regenerative growth is controlled by a homoeostat, then the intensity of the growth-stimulus at time t will be proportional to the difference between the final mass of the liver M_∞, and the mass, M_t, at time t. This model predicts that the mass, M_t, of the regenerating liver will follow the equation: $M_t = M_\infty(1 - e^{-\lambda t})$. Spencer and Coulombe (1966) have shown that the experimental results of Brues et al. (1936), covering the range $t = 1$ to $t = 12$ days, fit this equation with remarkable accuracy. The value of the constant λ was found to be 0·4 day^{-1}. These results agree quantitatively with our theory of growth-control by central elements.

Experiments of Czeizel et al. (1962) are of great importance to our thesis. They found that liver regeneration in the moderately-irradiated (500 R) partially-hepatectomised animal is arrested, but can be restored by injections of normal bone marrow. When the injected bone marrow is also irradiated, it fails to restore liver regeneration. Bone marrow therefore contains a factor, or factors, that are essential to regenerative growth in the heavily-irradiated animal: because they are destroyed by moderate doses (500 R) of ionising radiation, they almost certainly depend on cell division. These results are strikingly consistent with our theory, as are parallel findings concerning the effect of hind-limb shielding on heavily-irradiated mice. It is well known that a mouse will survive a normally supra-lethal dose of ionising radiation, provided only one hind limb is shielded from the radiation. Evidently the bone marrow in one hind limb contains a sufficient number and variety of growth-control cells to regenerate the vital tissues heavily damaged by radiation. Further supporting evidence along these lines is described in Chapter 10.

Most of the above experiments concern either the prevention of normal growth, or the restoration of the growth of artificially-reduced organs to their normal size. Extending the argument, we ought to be able to override the homoeostatic controls, and, by the suitable *addition* of appropriate lymphoid and/or myeloid growth-control tissue to an animal, we should be able to increase growth beyond its normal limits. Some remarkable experiments by Flaks (1967) have attained this aim. By injecting syngeneic thymic tissue into 3- to 5-day-old mice, and then by repeating these intra-peritoneal injections at fortnightly intervals, she was able to induce a marked increase in the general body size of the treated animals.

Horton (1967) concludes that the hair growth cycle in CBA mice is under systemic, and not local control, and other evidence we have reviewed elsewhere (Burch and Burwell 1965) tells a similar story: the normal growth of an organ is in part, at least, under central (systemic) control.

CAN WE HAVE ABSOLUTELY TRUE SCIENTIFIC LAWS?

There can be little doubt that premise (ii) is valid. No serious dispute is likely to arise regarding the truth of the other three premises. The argument developed from these empirical foundations is a simple one, and so are the conclusions. We have therefore to take seriously the almost sacrilegious possibility that we can have a scientific law that is non-trivial, and non-tautologous, but which is absolutely true because of 'biological necessity'. Complex organisms necessitate a form of growth-control in which common genes code for an MCP and its cognate TCF.

Happily, specific instances of the general law are eminently testable by experiment. Amino acid sequence analysis is still a formidable procedure, in more ways than one, but sooner or later it will be possible to isolate and purify MCPs and their cognate TCFs, and to find whether the corresponding polypeptides have the same amino acid sequence. As many as 7 genes may be involved in the synthesis of the protein component of these macromolecules (see next chapter), and if the structure of immunoglobulins is any guide, these genes may determine the sequence of around 7×100 amino acids.

Hence, if we found by experiment that 700 or so amino acid residues of polypeptide chains of an MCP appeared in the same sequence as those in the cognate TCF, we could conclude, with near certainty, that the same genes were involved in the coding of both MCP and TCF proteins. Such a demonstration – repeated for many MCP–TCF combinations – would constitute effective empirical 'proof' of our identity theory, which, so far, rests mainly on arguments from indirect evidence. Mainly but not entirely, because following the pioneering experiments of Medawar (1946), it is now well-established that leucocytes, and specifically lymphocytes, carry histocompatibility antigens, which form a part of the complex TCFs. This property is proving valuable in the selection of donors for tissue and organ transplantation (Amos *et al.* 1966). However, it has yet to be shown directly that growth-control lymphocytes carry antigens characteristic of their target tissue.

Verification of the MCP–TCF protein identity principle would be valuable, not only for practical transplantation studies, but also for theoretical biology. In the first place it would confirm a prediction, but beyond that, the principle could be put to use as an axiom in a deductive, and therefore rigorous if perhaps limited, biology of multi-tissue organisms. When combined with other axioms including the constancy in the number of growth-control stem cells during postnatal life, and the statistical law (Chapter 3) describing gene transitions in these cells, we could deduce the kinetical laws of the initiation of forbidden-clones in autoaggressive disease.

By now the alert and sceptical reader will have noticed one important omission from our scheme. When the efferent MCP and the afferent TCF are both humoral, how does the control system distinguish between them? (When the efferent MCP is cellular – carried by a small lymphocyte – and the afferent TCF is humoral, then no difficulty of principle arises, because these are different types of structure.) If MCPs and TCFs consisted of identical assemblies of polypeptide chains – and nothing else – then the growth-control system could never function because some distinction must exist between effectors and affectors. We have concluded that the distinction resides in the non-protein components of the molecules (Burch and Burwell 1965; Burch 1968a). Humoral MCPs are perhaps α_2-macroglobulins (at least, in some instances), and these proteins are complexed with carbohydrates; secreted TCFs are the humoral versions of histocompatibility antigens, and these are complexed mainly with lipids. Thus: *protein identity in MCPs and cognate TCFs provides for mutual recognition, while non-identity, of the non-protein components, provides for discrimination.*

FURTHER ASPECTS OF GROWTH-CONTROL

Our synthesis of Burnet's concept of disturbed-tolerance auto-immunity, with Burwell's ideas concerning growth-control, immediately explains why the number (L) of cells at somatic mutational risk in autoaggressive disease is constant throughout postnatal life. In Chapter 2, I pointed out that in a negative-feedback control of growth, the central part of the system has to contain a stable comparator to 'measure' the size of the target tissue, and to 'decide' whether it is too big or too small. With hindsight, it is difficult to see how, in a biological system, the growth-control comparator could consist of anything other than a fixed number of cells. We can be fairly confident, therefore, that autoaggressive diseases conforming to the biological model of Chapter 4, are initiated by somatic gene mutations in growth-control (comparator) stem cells.

Comments on other features of the growth-control mechanism may be appropriate at this point.

In Chapter 2, I followed Osgood in making the important, and often ignored distinction, between symmetrical and asymmetrical cell-division. From our general theory, it follows that the stimuli to these different forms of mitosis must themselves be different: symmetrical mitotis is promoted by centrally-derived MCPs, and asymmetrical mitosis must be homoeostatically governed by 'peripheral' or local factors. The use of a positive mitogenic stimulus (the effector MCP) to promote symmetrical mitosis implies that, in an organised tissue, cells are normally inhibited from undergoing this type of cell division. What then is the basis of inhibition? Following Swann (1957, 1958) we have argued that the normal contact relation between cells of a similar differentiation (that is, between TCFs of contiguous cells) is responsible for the inhibition of symmetrical mitosis (Burch and Burwell 1965). When this contact is broken – as in wounds and in tissue culture – mitosis proceeds in cells that are at the edge of the wound, and at the growing perimeter of the cultured tissue. (Malignant cells lack this capacity to inhibit mitosis in contiguous malignant cells: their TCFs are defective, and the mutual contact between 'mutant TCFs' evidently fails to establish those metabolic pathways that normally maintain the resting, or non-dividing state of the cell (Burch 1963b; Burch and Burwell 1965).) Furthermore, the TCF–TCF contact between similar non-malignant cells will be specific in character, and it will be maintained through London self-recognition forces. This is the phenomenon of *specific cellular adhesiveness* (Weiss 1958; Coman 1961; Abercrombie and Ambrose 1962) in which cells of a similar differentiation in tissue culture, on making contact with one another, remain in contact. The re-establishment of the correct functional nerve connections, following the experimental cutting of the optic nerve tract in fish, must also depend upon mutual TCF–TCF recognition between the regenerating axon and the surface of the post-synaptic cell. *Contact inhibition* (Abercrombie and Ambrose 1962) – in which the movement of wandering non-malignant cells in culture is arrested when similar cells make contact with one another – should also depend upon the change in cytoplasmic metabolism produced by TCF–TCF interaction. The defect in the TCFs of cancer cells can therefore explain why these cells usually exhibit neither contact inhibition, nor specific cellular adhesiveness. On this view, the malignant properties of the cancer cell arise from defective TCFs, which in turn, are produced in part by mutant genes and/or oncogenic viruses. Intensive investigation of the structure and function of cell membranes should therefore be relevant to the problems of malignant, as well as regenerative and normal growth.

7. A 'NEW' KIND OF MUTATION?
GENETIC AND BIOLOGICAL CONSEQUENCES

'A theory is the more impressive, the greater the simplicity of its premises is, the more different kinds of things it relates, and the more extended is its area of applicability.'

Albert Einstein, 1949

Biochemists and molecular biologists have made us familiar with the concept of 'point' mutation. In this type of gene change, a single base-pair is usually either altered (by a transition or transversion) or deleted. As we shall see below, this kind of mutation is unlikely to initiate autoaggressive disease.

EVIDENCE CONCERNING MUTATIONS

Somatic mutation-rates commonly show a 2 : 1 sex ratio ($k_F = 2k_M$). I attribute this to somatic mutation of an X-linked gene in growth-control stem cells, and I argued in the previous chapter that genes predisposing to an 'autoimmune' disease (e.g. systemic lupus erythematosus) may themselves undergo somatic mutation. Consider a specific gene locus on the X-chromosome – say *Xa* – where either of 2 alleles – *Xa1* and *Xa2* – may be found. Suppose *Xa1* predisposes, with dominant effect, to a given autoaggressive disease. Then predisposed females will be either homozygous: *Xa1/Xa1*, or heterozygous: *Xa1/Xa2*. Predisposed males will be *Xa1/(Y)*. If somatic mutation of the *Xa1* allele constitutes an initiating event, we would expect its rate to be the same in heterozygous *Xa1/Xa2* females as in *Xa1* males, but to be twice as high in homozygous *Xa1/Xa1* females. In the entire population of predisposed females, the average rate of somatic mutation of the *Xa1* allele ought, therefore, to lie between these limits, depending on the proportion of heterozygotes to homozygotes. Although this argument should apply to many diseases, I have found no evidence for such an intermediate rate. The argument is therefore false.

91

We could resolve the contradiction by postulating that geno-typic $Xa1/Xa2$ females become *phenotypically* $Xa1/Xa1$ in their growth-control stem cells through some form of *directed transition* during embryogenesis (Burch and Burwell 1965). On this view, MCP–TCF X-linked genes have two relatively stable, but mutually exclusive states (e.g. $Xa1$ or $Xa2$), and during embryogenesis, an induction mechanism converts one state, (e.g. $Xa2$) into the other (e.g. $Xa1$). Certain genes in other species appear to exist in fairly stable alternative states, as in paramutation (Brink 1960), and related phenomena (McClin-tock 1956; Dawson and Smith-Keary 1963; Finger and Heller 1964).

From studies of the familial aggregation of autoaggressive disease, we can distinguish *only two alleles* of an X-linked or an autosomal predisposing gene (Burch 1964a,b,c, 1966a; Burch and Rowell 1965a,b). Furthermore, the frequency of a pre-disposing allele calculated from such studies is usually high – often between 0·2 and 0·8 – and therefore indicative of genetic polymorphism.

Radiobiological findings are also germane to our inquiry. Extensive experiments have been carried out with mice to assess the sensitivity of each of seven genes (determining visible characters) to the mutagenic action of ionising radiation (see Russell 1964, 1965). The estimated size of the target that is sensitive to these radiation-induced mutations – with a mole-cular weight $\sim 3 \times 10^5$ daltons – is similar to the total DNA content of a typical structural gene (Burch 1967b). In other words, a specific mutation of this type can be produced by a radiation 'hit' almost anywhere on the gene: it cannot be necessary to 'hit' a specific base, or base-pair. On the other hand, when certain mutations are induced in yeast with heavily-ionising radiations, the effective target area is roughly equiva-lent to $10\overset{\circ}{A} \times 10\overset{\circ}{A}$ – which approximates to the cross-section presented by a single base-pair (Mortimer *et al.* 1965).

If mature post-meiotic germ cells in mice are irradiated, and if only one of the two strands of the DNA of a structural gene is 'hit', producing a point mutation, we would normally expect that about one-half of the cells of the inheritor would carry the mutation, while the remainder would be wild-type.

A visible character would usually show a mosaic pattern, rather than a whole-body effect.

Russell (1964) obtained no indication that 'mosaic mutations' are induced when mature germ cells are irradiated, although mosaicism is occasionally seen in the offspring both of irradiated and unirradiated animals. Hence, if the primary mutagenic event changes, say, a base on only one strand of DNA, then a 'correction' or repair mechanism must work with about 100 per cent efficiency to change the mis-matched base on the anti-parallel strand of DNA, to the form that is complementary to the mutant base. Although DNA repair mechanisms have been demonstrated in other contexts, (see the review by Hanawalt and Haynes, 1967), it is improbable that they would consistently function with complete efficiency.

SUMMARY OF EVIDENCE TO BE EXPLAINED

(1) Somatic mutations initiating autoaggressive disease occur at a constant rate, m (measured per unit time, rather than per cell generation), which is independent of postnatal age and ordinary environments. (2) The high rates of somatic mutation at some loci in M cells ($m > 10^{-4}$ per year), and comparable rates for certain mutations in bacteria. (3) Indications from the mammalian and bacterial evidence that a unimolecular reaction mechanism might be involved. (4) At many MCP – TCF loci, only two alleles can be detected by the analysis of familial evidence for autoaggressive diseases. (5) The frequency of detectable predisposing alleles often lies between 0·2 and 0·8. (6) A directed change ('directed mutation') from one X-linked allele, to its alternative allele, might occur during embryogenesis. Such a change could make a genotypically heterozygous female, phenotypically homozygous at MCP – TCF loci in growth-control stem cells. (7) Gene changes initiating auto-aggressive disease convert an *identity* relation between protein components of an MCP and its cognate TCF, into a *complementary* and pathogenic relation between the primary autoantibody (the mutant MCP) and its related TCF. (8) The target size for the induction of this kind of gene transition by ionising radiation is roughly equivalent to the total DNA content of the gene. (9) Most, and perhaps all 'visible' mutations

induced by ionising radiation in post-meiotic germ cells in mice are whole-body, as opposed to mosaic in expression.

DNA STRAND-SWITCHING MUTATION

So far, only one solution has been proposed that is consistent with all these nine considerations: the random gene change initiating autoaggressive disorders involves a spontaneous

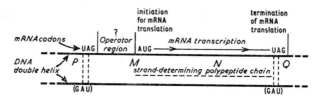

(i) *Left to Right mRNA transcription from upper strand of DNA double helix. Polypeptide chain product is encoded by MQ section of DNA strand.*

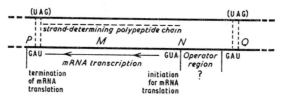

(ii) *Situation after DNA strand-switching "mutation" Right to Left mRNA transcription from N P section of lower DNA strand.*

Fig. 7.1   Possible arrangement of initiating (AUG) and terminating (UAG) codons at an MCP–TCF gene locus (Burch 1968a). The punctuating codons define a stretch PQ of DNA double helix that allows mRNA synthesis to occur by transcribing either strand of DNA. Normally, transcription occurs from one strand only (the informational strand), and the polypeptide chain product associates with the non-informational strand to prevent it being transcribed. Dissociation of the strand-determining polypeptide chain from the DNA, followed by transcription from the 'wrong' (formerly non-informational strand) is called a *DNA strand-switching* mutation. In (i), MQ is the informational stretch of DNA and in (ii), NP, on the anti-parallel strand, is the informational stretch. The phase shift of one base between the two strands is described in the text. The non-simultaneous exploitation of information from either strand of DNA is called *genetic dichotomy*. This scheme awaits experimental confirmation.

switch in messenger RNA (*m*RNA) transcription from the regular strand of DNA over to the base-paired, anti-parallel strand. (See Fig. 7.1.) We call this a DNA *strand-switching mutation* (Burch and Burwell 1965).

In the synthesis of many proteins, the DNA template of a cistron in the nucleus is first *transcribed* by the synthesis of a messenger RNA (*m*RNA) which is complementary to the informational strand of the double-stranded DNA. Messenger RNA is then *translated* in the cytoplasm (by the ribosome cum transfer-RNA system) into polypeptide chains. The direction of *m*RNA transcription from the DNA template, and the direction of translation of *m*RNA, are both polarised, and they proceed in the 5′ to 3′ direction of the sugar-phosphate backbone.

Some mechanism must determine which of the two strands of DNA is the informational strand available for *m*RNA transcription. For MCP–TCF genes, I envisage that the polypeptide chain product of a gene normally determines which of the two strands of the DNA duplex is available for *m*RNA transcription. It probably associates with the complementary, non-informational strand, to block *m*RNA transcription from it. Generally, this constitutes a self-locking device. In the course of mitosis, surplus DNA strand-selection polypeptide chains must be made available to complex with the non-informational strand of the newly replicated DNA, and to maintain the original gene expression.

If, however, the complex between DNA and the strand-determining polypeptide should dissociate, *m*RNA transcription from the hitherto non-informational strand of DNA would then become possible. After translation of the 'wrong' *m*RNA, the new polypeptide chain could then associate with the original, informational strand, to block *m*RNA transcription from it and to establish the mutation. Generally, the initial act of dissociation occurs spontaneously, but it can also be induced by extrinsic mutagens such as ionising radiation.

In embryogenesis, 'directed mutation' of a gene at an X-linked MCP–TCF locus in heterozygous females requires that the changeover from one DNA strand to its complement should be effected at one of the two homologous genes by a positive induction mechanism.

SOMATIC MUTATIONS AND CARCINOGENESIS

Validation of our DNA strand-switching idea would have an important consequence. Mutagens such as nitrous acid and hydroxylamine that can induce point mutations, will not necessarily induce strand-switching mutations. Other mutagens, such as ionising radiation can probably induce both forms of gene change. The lack of a consistent one-to-one correspondence between mutagenic and carcinogenic agents has been used to support objections to somatic mutation theories of carcinogenesis. If strand-switching mutations help to initiate malignant change – and this is distinctly possible – then such criticisms become irrelevant.

IMPLICATIONS OF DNA STRAND-SWITCHING THEORY.
SUPPORTING EVIDENCE

Support for the idea that a third strand or chain may be associated with double-stranded DNA is provided by the analysis (Burch 1967b) of experiments on radiation cytotoxicity. When the proliferative capacity of mammalian cells is destroyed by densely-ionising particles, the inactivating mechanism involves a triple energy-transfer from the ionising particle to a complex target. The radio-sensitive target has a total cross-sectional area approximating to that of the nucleus of the cell. The spacing between the triple energy-transfers (successive events) is in the region of 10 Å. (The outside diameter of the chromatid thread is about 30 Å.) Independent evidence indicates that nuclear DNA is the main target for this type of radiation action. Probably, two of the three 'dependent-type' energy transfers break the sugar-phosphate backbone of both strands of DNA, while the third may break another structure, which could be the DNA strand-determining polypeptide chain.

If a strand-switching mutation converts a protein identity relation between an MCP and its cognate TCF into a complementary relation (point (6) above), then from Fig. 7.2, we see that specific steric relations, of a broadly complementary nature, should exist between at least some amino acids and their related codons. These relations make possible a complementary fit between the strand-determining polypeptide chain and the bases of a suitably coiled non-informational DNA strand. They also cater for the change from the identity relation between the protein components of an MCP and its TCF to the complementary relation between the primary autoantibody ('mutant' MCP) and its target TCF.

The required specific steric relation between at least some amino acids and their codons is, perhaps, the most controversial feature of the proposal. Although several authors

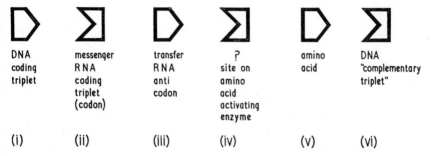

DNA coding triplet	messenger RNA coding triplet (codon)	transfer RNA anti codon	? site on amino acid activating enzyme	amino acid	DNA "complementary triplet"
(i)	(ii)	(iii)	(iv)	(v)	(vi)

Fig. 7.2 Broadly complementary stereochemical relations proposed for DNA-dependent protein synthesis (Burch 1966c). Those between (i) and (ii); (ii) and (iii); and (i) and (vi) are well established.

(Weinstein 1963; Nirenberg *et al.* 1965; Pelc 1965; Woese 1965) have suggested, for quite independent reasons, (universality of the genetic code; regularities in the code; correspondence between amino acid and base-triplet structures) that such a relation might exist, it has not yet been established. However, Woese *et al.* (1966) have demonstrated specific chemical interactions between amino acids and organic bases, and they conclude that the codon assignments of the genetic code reflect an underlying pairing between each codon and its associated amino acid. Furthermore, Leng and Felsenfeld (1966) have demonstrated preferential interactions of synthetic polylysine and polyarginine with specific base sequences of DNA.

The scheme illustrated in Fig. 7.2 also requires: (a) the *t*RNA anti-codon should be broadly complementary (as in Crick's (1966) 'wobble'-hypothesis) to its *m*RNA codon *and* to the amino acid recognition site on the amino acid activating enzyme (i.e. the aminoacyl *t*RNA synthetase); (b) because the recognition site on the activating enzyme should also be broadly complementary to its specific amino acid, the activated amino acid must be transported from this recognition site on the eynzyme to another site before the *t*RNA is encountered.

Crick's (1966) 'wobble' hypothesis has been confirmed for several codon-anti-codon pairs. Evidence for the view that the *t*RNA anti-codon also recognises the aminoacyl *t*RNA synthetase is still inconclusive (see Hayashi and Miura 1966, their literature review and, more recently, Brostoff and Ingram 1967). Fortunately for our scheme, it is now established that a *t*RNA complexes with its specific aminoacyl *t*RNA synthetase, in the absence of ATP and the related amino acid (Yarus and Berg 1967). Hence the steric relation postulated between (iii) and (iv) in Fig. 7.2 is reasonably well supported.

In many *in vitro* systems (see the review by Hayes 1967) *m*RNA transcription takes place from both strand of DNA – this is called 'symmetrical transcription'. Geiduschek *et al.* (1964) showed that denatured phage DNA supported symmetrical transcription, but on renaturation, it recovered the capacity to direct asymmetrical transcription; the exact conditions necessary for asymmetrical transcription were not determined. (Denaturation, which involves partial-to-complete separation of the two strands of the DNA double helix, may be expected to lead to the dissociation from the DNA of a strand-determining polypeptide chain.)

In bacteria (Margolin 1965; Sanderson 1965; Hartman *et al.* 1965; Beckwith and Signer 1966), and in phage λDNA (Cohen and Hurwitz 1967; K. Taylor *et al.* 1967), *m*RNA transcription occurs in one direction from certain regions of the genome – and therefore along one strand of DNA – while at other regions, transcription occurs in the opposite direction, and therefore from the complementary strand of DNA. Under *in vivo* conditions, specific signals evidently determine which of the two DNA strands is available for *m*RNA transcription in phage λ and in bacteria. It does not follow that the same kind of signals are effective in mammalian cells. Nevertheless, the evidence from these lower organisms shows there is nothing magical about one strand of DNA where *m*RNA transcription is concerned: a specific signal or mechanism selects one of the two strands as the informational strand for protein synthesis.

At some operons the 'clockwise' strand is selected, at other operons the 'anticlockwise' strand is made available.

In spite of these many promising indications, the experimental evidence and arguments in favour of DNA strand-switching mutations, and of DNA strand-selection, are on a less secure footing than those supporting the principles of protein identity (partial or complete), between MCPs and cognate TCFs. The geometry of the relation between the strand-determining polypeptide chain and the non-informational strand of DNA, presents the biggest stumbling-block, but a fuller understanding of the structure of the chromosome, and of the distinction between euchromatin and heterochromatin, may clarify these current obscurities. Proteins constitute the greater part of the bulk of chromosomes but their function remains to be elucidated.

PREDICTIONS OF DNA STRAND-SWITCHING THEORY

The theory makes two exact predictions. Firstly, the amino acid sequence of the portion MN of the 'non-mutant' polypeptide chain should be related to the sequence of the portion NM of its 'complementary' or mutant chain, through Watson-Crick A–T, G–C base-pairing, and the genetic code (See Fig. 7.1.) Because of the regularities in the code, and the nature of two terminating codons, UAA and UAG (Weigert and Garen 1965; Brenner, Stretton and Kaplan 1965) we suggested (Burch and Burwell 1965) that a strand-switching mutation is likely to be accompanied by a phase-shift. That is to say, if the base sequence on one strand of DNA is represented by ... Z, ABC, DEF ... then the complementary sequence on the anti-parallel strand should be represented by: F_c, $E_c D_c C_c$, $B_c A_c Z_c$, where the commas demarcate 'DNA codons', and A_c is the base complementary to A, etc. Secondly, the direction of mRNA transcription will be reversed by a strand-switching event. Although these two predictions are precise, the technical difficulties in the way of testing them are still somewhat daunting.

Allowing for the phase shift, the 'complement' of the initiating codon AUG, is AU(Z), where the base (Z) will be complementary to the base preceding AUG. Terminating codons

UAA and UAG both have UA(Z) as their 'complements' and hence when (Z) is A or G, these triplets can serve as terminating codons on the 'complementary strand' of mRNA (see Fig. 7.1). The four codons CGU, CGC, CGA and CGG all code for arginine, and so do their 'complementary' codons; similarly, the four codons GCU, GCC, GCA and GCG code for alanine, and so do their complementary codons. In these instances (and two others) an amino acid is identical with its 'complement'.

NON-SEGREGATING MUTATIONS

Non-segregating mutations observed in bacteria (Kubitschek 1964) are analogous to 'whole-body' mutations seen in higher organisms: both daugher cells inherit the mutation induced in the progenitor cell. Hence the strand-switching mechanism could be relevant to this form of mutation in bacteria.

GENE REGULATION

In bacteria, and their phages, it appears that a specific inter-action between a repressor protein and the operator region of an operon, blocks mRNA transcription from the subsequent cistrons (structural genes) lying within the operon (Ptashne 1967). To account for the affinity of the repressor for the operator, it seems likely that the amino acids, or prosthetic groups of the repressor protein, interact specifically with the DNA bases of the appropriate operator. The repressor-operator interaction in bacteria, may parallel the mechanism of DNA strand-selection at MCP–TCF genes in multi-tissue organisms.

CELLULAR DIFFERENTIATION AND EMBRYOGENESIS

Many important properties of cells in higher organisms are closely, and perhaps indissolubly interrelated: (i) the antigenic (TCF) specificity of the plasma membrane and endoplasmic reticulum; (ii) morphology; and (iii) physiological, including biochemical function. We have to determine which, if any, of these three properties is 'cause', and which is 'effect'. It is very difficult to imagine how (ii) or (iii), which characterise the mature cell in the developed organism, could precede the induction of specific genes coding for the TCF. On the other hand, because the differentiation of a cell is fundamentally a matter of differential gene expression, the prior induction of TCF genes could then be responsible for the remaining properties of the cell. By a direct or indirect mechanism, TCF proteins, or their sub-units, could determine the general pattern of gene activity in differentiated cells. However, this general pattern has to allow several alternative metabolic and functional states. In an organised tissue, external factors such as MCPs, can interact with the cell to switch metabolic pathways from the resting phase, to those leading to symmetrical or asymmetrical mitosis. Conceivably, special non-TCF 'differentiating genes' could be repressed or depressed during organogenesis, in parallel with TCF genes, but the lack of disjunction between (i) and the other properties of the differentiated cell makes this an uneconomical hypothesis.

The concept of cellular differentiation that emerges from this discussion differs slightly from the traditional view, which is based more on histological than on immunological (TCF) criteria. In a cell line such as the erythrocytic, where late or 'mature' cells have a highly-specialised function, differences between the stem cells, intermediate, and late cells, are probably governed by changes in the protein, and/or non-protein components of the TCF. This change in gene expression will be produced, directly or indirectly, by the stimulus for asymmetrical mitosis. Cells of the growth-control series will also exhibit corresponding changes as maturation proceeds from the bone marrow stem cells, via the intermediate, to the final effector forms.

In view of the great specificity of TCFs, and the comparable specificity of cellular differentiation, appreciable dissociation between these two key properties in normal cells is unlikely. I therefore propose that the *induction of TCF genes is the primary step in cellular differentiation.*

Because some or all of the polypeptide chains of an MCP are identical with those of its cognate TCF, each MCP–TCF element may derive from a common precursor cell during embryogenesis. This common (postzygotic) precursor divides asymmetrically to give one daughter cell (M) to act as a progenitor for growth-control stem cells, and another daughter cell (T), to act as a progenitor for the target tissue.

Differences between M and T cells might reside in the non-protein components of the MCP and TCF respectively. Because the number of growth-control stem cells in any element is probably fixed before birth, a single specific M cell may give rise to a fixed number (L) of descendant growth-control stem cells. This exact control of the number (L) of stem cells would appear to require a serial 'counting' mechanism, linked to DNA replication and/or some other feature of cell division.

STRUCTURE OF MCPs AND TCFs

The number of genetically distinctive polypeptide components making up a given MCP or TCF is of great interest, and the evidence from autoaggressive disease provides a guide to the complexity of these proteins. If the value of r in the equations of Chapter 4 generally represents the number of strand-switching mutations per stem cell (as it probably does) then this can be as high as 6 autosomal events (myasthenia gravis), but it might be as high as 12 (spontaneous trochanteric fractures of the femur). Assuming that 2 autosomal events may affect both homologous genes at a specific locus, then the minimum number of loci involved in the synthesis of at least some TCFs, is 3 autosomal and 1 X-linked, but it might be as high as (or indeed, higher than) 6 autosomal and 1 X-linked. However Y-linked histocompatibility antigens are also found in males, and the importance of both X- and Y-linked factors in sex-differentiation is discussed below.

It seems unlikely that the induction of a complete set of MCP–TCF genes in a precursor cell is accomplished in one step. A sequential programme, proceeding from the primitive to the most mature state seems more in keeping with the phenomena of embryogenesis. We are told, after all, that ontogeny mirrors phylogeny.

To solve the 'tissue code' we shall have to specify fully the composition and structure of TCFs for every distinctive tissue. When we consider the ferocious complexity of even a single TCF, and when we reflect that one man may have as many as 10^8 of these enigmatic structures, the challenge presented by the tissue code will surely intimidate even the most fanatical devotees of automation and computerisation. But it might be wise to get this little problem out of the way before embarking on genetic engineering and similar conceits. For some time to come, I suspect we shall have to reconcile ourselves to an incomplete inventory and description of TCFs.

Useful pointers to the simpler features of TCFs are provided by transplantation experiments, the genetics of autoaggressive disease, and the positive and negative associations between such diseases (see Chapter 10). Evidence of this latter kind can show whether TCF polypeptides are shared or not shared by different tissues. So far, I have found no indication that X-linked factors are shared by tissues that can be distinguished at the ordinary level, and hence at least one of the antigens that distinguishes one tissue from another at this level may be coded by an X-linked gene. Evidence from dental caries (Chapter 8) indicates that odontoblast tissue in teeth, which is homogeneous by ordinary histological criteria, is actually a mosaic compounded of many antigenically-distinctive groups of cells.

EMBRYOLOGY. THE PRIMARY TASK

If I am correct in suggesting that the induction of MCP–TCF genes occurs serially, step by step, then the primary task in embryology is the elucidation of the mechanism of gene induction. Is information selected sequentially from the DNA 'tape'? Is this accomplished by the serial movement of an inducer, stepping along one cistron at a time, at each cycle of DNA replication? (This is a modern version of the preformationist concept.) Or does intercellular interaction produce repression and derepression of genes through the kind of regulatory (operon) mechanism found in bacteria (Jacob and Monod 1961)? In other words, is an epigenetic process involved? Or, more plausibly, are both types of mechanism involved?

To answer these questions we shall have to analyse the antigenic composition of plasma membranes at successive stages of embryogenesis, and to correlate MCP–TCF gene activity with genetic switching mechanisms.

GENETIC POLYMORPHISM AND SEX DIFFERENTIATION. THEORY
OF GENETIC DICHOTOMY

Individuality, both of appearance and behaviour, is something
with which we are all familiar. Only monozygotic twins can
show a virtually identical appearance. However, even the
gross morphological differences between men and women
have not been adequately explained.

By definition, the overall morphology of an organism is the
expression of the number, size, shape, and arrangement of its
component parts – cells and extra-cellular materials. In our
theory, the size and shape of a cell is determined, directly or
indirectly, by its TCF and its contact with neighbouring cells
and structures such as basement membranes; the orientation
of one cell to its neighbours is determined by TCF–TCF
interaction. Growth itself, beyond a certain stage of embryogenesis, is mainly determined by MCP–TCF interactions.
Because the unit macromolecule of each of the numerous
MCP–TCF elements in an individual may be made up of at
least seven genetically-distinctive sections of polypeptide chains;
and because MCP–TCF genetic loci appear generally to have
two distinguishable alleles, it is scarcely surprising that we are
not all alike.

It follows from our theory of growth-control and cellular
differentiation that the morphological and functional differences
between the sexes ought to derive from the contributions of
sex-linked genes to MCPs and TCFs. Although qualitative
differences at the ordinary chemical level between the sexes
may be undetectable (Mittwoch 1967), immunological differences, at the level of transplantation (TCF) antigens, are readily
demonstrated, and they support our prediction. Eichwald and
Silmser (1955) pointed to the possible presence of Y-linked
transplantation antigens in male mice and their suggestion was
subsequently confirmed (see, for example, Billingham et al.
1965). Bailey (1963) was the first to demonstrate X-linked
histoincompatibility antigens in mice.

Our own analyses of the age-patterns and genetics of autoaggressive diseases give frequent indications of X-linkage and
occasional ones of Y-linkage in the synthesis of MCP–TCF
polypeptides. Because both homologous X-linked MCP genes

are probably active in the growth-control stem cells of normal XX females, the morphological differences between them, and individuals with Turner's (XO) syndrome, can be accounted for. A gene dosage effect at X-linked MCP loci may also contribute to the differences between normal males and females, and between normal males and individuals with Klinefelter's (XXY) syndrome; the excessive height of XYY individuals is not surprising.

Both the existence, and the preservation of innumerable polymorphic characters within a species are predictable consequences of our theory, although they embarrass orthodox geneticists. Thus, Neel and Salzano (1967) comment: 'Without question, the focal problem in human population genetics today is to understand the biological significance of the many polymorphisms now recognised – as well as those almost certainly awaiting discovery. If, on the one hand, they are maintained by selection, then, as genetic loads have been formulated the *burden* that polymorphisms would appear to impose on a population is of such a magnitude as to require reconsideration of load theory. If, on the other hand, the polymorphisms are neutral, it is difficult to understand the occurrence of *specific* polymorphisms in such a variety of populations (as opposed to the accumulation at each locus of many mutant genes because of simple mutation pressure). Between these two polarizations there are of course many intermediate possibilities.'

On strand-switching theory, if each of the two 'complementary' polypeptide chains – the products of the complementary strands of DNA at an MCP–TCF locus – gives rise to a viable phenotype, then spontaneous DNA strand-switching in the germ-cell line will always maintain a minimum of two alleles at that locus. If the rates of the spontaneous transitions ($a_1 \rightleftharpoons a_2$) between two complementary alleles are equal, and if selection pressures against both homozygotes are equal – including the special case of zero or neutral selection pressures – then in a large random breeding population both alleles will always attain the equilibrium frequency of 0·5. Neither allele is 'wild-type' and neither is 'mutant'. We have referred to the (non-simultaneous) utilisation of the information from both strands of DNA, as *genetic dichotomy* (Burch and Burwell 1965).

8

Should a point mutation occur in the common section of DNA (MN, Fig. 7.1), and should the polypeptide chains associated with both mutant strands of DNA give rise to viable phenotypes, then eventually strand-switching will give rise to an additional pair of alleles. They may or may not be distinguishable from the original alleles at the ordinary (non-molecular) clinical, or genetic (familial) levels of analysis.

HETEROZYGOUS FITNESS (OVER-DOMINANCE)

From studies of sex- and age-patterns and familial and twins evidence, we have found that predisposition to autoaggressive disease often involves homozygosity at at least one autosomal locus; the heterozygote is not predisposed (Burch 1964b,c; 1966a; 1968b; Burch and Rowell 1965b, 1968). When the auto-aggressive disease impairs reproductive fitness – as it often does – heterozygous fitness is accounted for.

INTERGENIC RECOMBINATION AT MCP–TCP LOCI

Despite its central importance in genetics, no interpretation of the mechanism of recombination has won general acceptance. However, there are many indications that inter- and intra-genic recombination are different phenomena. The concept of *genetic dichotomy* leads to an uncomplicated theory of intergenic recombination at MCP–TCF loci (Burch 1966c).

Suppose one allele at a gene locus on the chromatid corresponds to *m*RNA transcription from one strand of DNA. Suppose the homologous allele on the other chromatid corresponds to *m*RNA transcription from the anti-parallel strand of DNA. If during meiosis an exchange of DNA strand-determining polypeptide chains occurs between these paired homologous genes after DNA synthesis, this will effect intergenic recombination. (See Fig. 7.3.)

THE LYON HYPOTHESIS

According to Lyon (1961) one of the X-chromosomes in the cells of XX females is inactivated during an early stage of embryogenesis to form the Barr body: the choice between the paternally-derived, and the maternally-derived X-chromosome

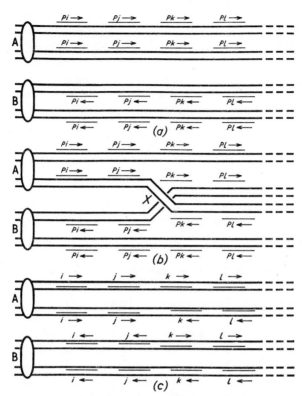

Fig. 7.3 Possible mechanism for intergenic recombination at MCP–TCF loci. (a) Homologous pairing of the sister chromatids A and B. Tetrad at the end of DNA synthesis. Strand-determining polypeptide chains ($pi\rightarrow$, $pi\leftarrow$, etc.) have not yet associated with their stretch of DNA. (b) Random chiasma formation at point X. After synapse formation, the DNA duplexes acquire adjacent strand-determining polypeptide chains. (c) Completion of recombination. A reciprocal exchange of polypeptide chains $pk\rightarrow$, $pl\rightarrow$ . . . and $pk\leftarrow$, $pl\leftarrow$ . . . between an A and a B chromatid has been effected.

is supposed to be made randomly, and, once established, the pattern of inactivation is then transmitted without change to descendant cells. Grüneberg (1966, 1967) has examined many phenotypes at the tissue (multi-cellular) level, both in mice and in women, who are heterozygous for known X-linked traits. He has found no evidence to support Lyon's postulate that the inactivation of one of the two X-chromosomes is made randomly Where the heterozygotes show phenotypic effects at the tissue level, mosaic patterning is regular, rather than random.

According to our hypothesis, all the cells of a single element of a tissue mosaic, as well as their growth-control cells, descend from a single precursor cell in which the X-linked gene directing the synthesis of a specific MCP–TCF polypeptide is induced during embryogenesis. In females who are genotypically heterozygous $(Xa1/Xa2)$ at an X-linked MCP–TCF gene locus, the induction mechanism selects equivalent strands of DNA, at both homologous genes, so that the precursor cell becomes phenotypically homozygous (say, $Xa1/Xa1$). Thus the precursor cell in females always shows similar alleles, with the same direction of mRNA transcription at this X-linked MCP–TCF locus, although at non-MCP–TCF loci, the maternally- and paternally-derived chromosomes may carry different alleles.

The precursor cell divides asymmetrically to form two groups of cells: the mesenchymal growth-control stem cells (M) and the related target tissue cells (T). I conclude that, in M cells of females, both homologous X-linked MCP genes are active, because both are at mutational risk in the initiation of auto-aggressive disease (Burch 1963c). Consequently, we should not see Barr body formation in these cells, which are located mainly in the bone marrow. This prediction agrees strikingly with observation: Barr bodies are not seen in the bone marrow (Hamerton 1964). In most target tissue cells, however, the inactivation of one X-chromosome occurs with Barr body formation, and at this stage the choice as to which chromosome is inactivated might, in principle at least, be made randomly. Because both X-chromosomes carry the same allele at the TCF locus, (neglecting the possibility of point mutations) all cells in a given tissue element will have the same TCF. But if X-linked genes in these cells code for one or more non-TCF proteins, then two types of cell may be distinguishable: those with the active paternally-derived, and those with the active maternally-derived X-chromosome. These two types of cell might therefore be distributed randomly within the tissue element.

All complex tissues such as epidermis, bone, and even the liver parenchyma, will be mosaics with multiple elements arranged in a systematic pattern. Many elements of a given tissue may share a common X-linked TCF locus, and in genotypically heterozygous females some elements may display one allele $(Xa1)$, while others show the alternative allele $(Xa2)$.

The choice will be made during embryogenesis by the 'directed-mutation' induction mechanism, which will be genetically-determined. When a tissue consists of a single element only, as is perhaps the case with erythrocytes, then only one X-linked TCF antigen will be found in heterozygous females. This prediction is borne out where the Xg blood factor is concerned: erythrocytes of heterozygous females are phenotypically X$g(a+)$.

However, the enzyme glucose-6-phosphate dehydrogenase (G6PD) is said to be coded by an X-linked gene, and, as the result of Barr-body formation in nucleated target cells, we might expect heterozygous females to exhibit some cells with normal enzyme activity, and others with deficient activity. This form of mosaicism is seen in the erythrocytes of females who are heterozygous for glucose-6-phosphate dehydrogenase deficiency (see for example Davidson et al. 1963; Gartler et al. 1966; and Kosower et al. 1967).

At first sight these findings, when taken in conjunction with the non-mosaic distribution of the Xg antigen, appear to provide direct proof of the foregoing scheme. Unfortunately, other evidence favours a different interpretation. Males, with only one X-chromosome, can show mild G6PD deficiency accompanied by so-called 'pseudomosaicism' in their erythrocytes. This phenomenon has been attributed to red-cell ageing (Schneer 1967). If this view is correct, another form of red-cell ageing, producing loss or destruction of G6PD activity, might account for the 'genuine' mosaicism in heterozygous females. The strongest – though still inconclusive – evidence against the random inactivation of an X-linked G6PD gene in females, is provided by a study of twins (Brewer et al. 1967). In Negro female twins heterozygous for G6PD deficiency, intrapair differences in red cell G6PD activity and mosaicism were much smaller in monozygotic than in dizygotic twins. Brewer et al. (1967) incline to the hypothesis that X-chromosome inactivation is genetically-, and not randomly-determined.

Clearly, the evidence for G6PD deficiency must be scrutinised with special care. But on the present showing, inactivation of one X chromosome in the target cells of XX females is unlikely to involve a random process. Whereas most intrinsic *pathological* changes include a random element, the exquisite precision of *developmental* phenomena derives from a rigidly deterministic mechanism.

In the Hiroshima population studied by Freedman *et al.* (1968), the prevalence of diabetes mellitus was much higher in men than in women, for all ages above 20 years. In Western populations (see, for example, Fig. 4.7) women are usually more prone to diabetes than men. However, in the last century diabetes was more common in men, and the sex-ratio (M/F) for standardised mortality rates for diabetes in England and Wales, changed from 2 in 1861, to 1·2 in 1911, and to 0·8 in 1936 (Fitzgerald 1967). Since 1953, standardised mortality ratios have been increasing slightly in men, and staying more-or-less constant in women (Registrar General 1965). Similar trends have been found among white, Massachusetts residents, at the Joslin Clinic, Boston (Hirohata *et al.* 1967). In 1939, the number of new male cases diagnosed at the Clinic was 210, and of female cases 284, giving a crude sex-ratio (M/F) of 0·74. The corresponding ratio progressively increased to 1·04 (447/433) in 1959.

That is to say, the X-linked factor predisposing (with autosomal factors) to diabetes mellitus, can have a recessive expression in some countries, and at certain periods, to give an excess of predisposed males; but at other times, and/or in other countries, its expression is dominant, giving an excess of predisposed females.

Our theory of genetic dichotomy offers a straightforward interpretation of this variability in the sex-ratio of predisposed individuals (Burch and Burwell 1965). Suppose the predisposing X-linked allele is *XD1*, and the alternative allele at the same locus, corresponding to transcription from DNA in the opposite direction, is *XD2*. When dominance is observed, genotypically heterozygous females (*XD1/XD2*) generally become phenotypically *XD1/XD1* in precursor growth-control cells during embryogenesis. When X-linked recessiveness is found, the directed strand-switching mechanism generally converts the precursor cell in the heterozygous female to the non-predisposing *XD2/XD2* phenotype.

The choice between the alternative transitions $(XD_1 \rightarrow XD_2;$ $XD_2 \rightarrow XD_1)$, may depend on one or more products of particular autosomal MCP–TCF alleles. Hence, variation in the sex-ratio of predisposition is likely to be determined by changes in allelic frequencies at autosomal loci. In turn, these frequencies will be affected by the 'forward' and 'backward' rates of strand-switching mutation at MCP–TCF genes in germ cells, and by selection pressures.

ORIGIN AND EVOLUTION OF MCP–TCF GENES

The functional demands made on MCP–TCF proteins encourage speculation concerning the evolutionary origin of the genes that code for them. According to our theory of genetic dichotomy, the transcription of an MCP–TCF gene in one direction corresponds to one major allele, and, with strand-switching, the transcription of the gene in the opposite direction corresponds to the other major allele. Because poly-peptide chains associated with both directions of transcription

POSSIBLE ORIGIN OF MCP–TCF GENE

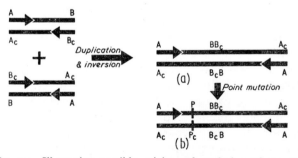

Fig. 7.4 Illustrating possible origin and evolution of growth-control genes. AB represents one strand (5' to 3') of the DNA double-helix, and B_cA_c represents the anti-parallel strand. Bases A_c and B_c are complementary to A and B respectively. In (a), duplication and inversion have occurred. The information in the top strand, ABB_cA_c reads the same as that from the bottom, anti-parallel strand. (b) If a point mutation occurs at P, and if it is 'incorporated' either through semi-conservative replication or 'repair' mechanisms in the anti-parallel strand at P_c (where the base P_c is complementary to P), then the information $APBB_cA_c$ from the top strand, differs from $ABB_cP_cA_c$ from the lower anti-parallel strand.

have to serve the same general purpose, the most primitive MCP–TCF gene probably produced the same polypeptide chain when read in 'forward' or 'backward' directions. Gene duplication, accompanied by inversion could secure this (Fig. 7.4a), and the information along the 'top' strand of DNA (ABB_cA_c) reads the same as that along the 'bottom' strand. Subsequent mutation of a base at P, accompanied by a change in the complementary base at P_c, could then cause the two sequences: $APBB_cA_c$ (top strand), and $ABB_cP_cA_c$ (bottom strand), to differ (Fig. 7.4b). Provided both new 'mutant' polypeptide chains resulting from these DNA base changes are acceptable (in the functional and evolutionary senses) the mutant genes could become established. Replication of such genes, followed by further viable point mutations, could introduce variations essential to evolutionary change. Polypeptide chains serving similar but not identical functions in the TCFs of advanced organisms, might be expected to have substantial regions of homology, and to differ only slightly in their amino acid sequences after the manner of the small differences observed in the 'variable' N-terminal halves of immunoglobulin 'light' (λ or κ) chains.

Summarising, if the first MCP–TCF gene gave the same message for both directions of transcription, it yielded no polymorphisms. This source of diversity, indispensable to evolutionary adaptation, had to await point mutation. A most important form of variation was provided by the first point mutation that gave acceptable amino acid substitutions in the two polypeptide chains, resulting from both directions of transcription. An increase in the number and specificity of MCP–TCF genes per genome led to further polymorphisms. Proceeding along the phylogenetic scale, organisational complexity depends, not only on the total *number* of distinctive MCP–TCF genes, but also on the distinctive *combinations* of genes contributing to the synthesis of each MCP–TCF macromolecule.

ELEGANCE AND CORRECTNESS

I think it is not unfair to claim that the hypotheses of DNA strand-switching and genetic dichotomy offer elegant solutions to some outstanding problems in genetics. Although Gamow

(1967) . . . 'quite agrees with Dirac in his conviction that if a theory is elegant, it must be correct . . .' I presume we are not intended to interpret this statement too literally. When observations can be explained in terms of several hypotheses, then in the absence of bias we prefer to adopt the most elegant or economical one. But in empirical science, a main pre-occupation is the invention of crucial tests that will enable us to choose between theoretical alternatives – elegant or other-wise. Proof of the DNA strand-switching hypothesis of mutation will clearly have to await amino acid sequence analysis of 'complementary' polypeptide chains, and/or the demonstration of a reversal in the direction of transcription.

8. ANATOMICAL DISTRIBUTION OF DISEASE

'Now if pathology is nothing but physiology with obstacles, and diseased life nothing but healthy life interfered with by all manner of external and internal influences, then pathology too must be referred back to the cell.'

Rudolph Virchow, 1855. (L. J. Rather's translation)

One of the most intriguing and one of the most neglected features of disease is its anatomical distribution. Arthritis may affect many or only one of a patient's joints, while the others remain normal. If we examine a cross-section of the shaft of an aged femur, we may find marked porosity in say two quadrants, and a normal bone structure in the other two (Atkinson and Weatherall 1967). Burkitt's lymphoma of the jaws shows a very complicated but non-random distribution (Adatia 1966). Either, or both sides of the mandible may be affected while the maxilla remains normal. The reverse situation is also found, but both maxilla and mandible are involved in some cases. In still other patients, all four quadrants are involved (see Chapter 11). Examples of the specific site distribution of disease, especially from dermatology and neurology, could be multiplied almost indefinitely.

Why should one part of a given kind of tissue undergo proliferative or degenerative change, while another and even an adjacent part is quite commonly spared? Why should a lesion on the left be accompanied by a symmetrical lesion on the right in some patients, but not in others? These are the fascinating questions we shall discuss in this chapter.

DISTRIBUTION OF DENTAL CARIES IN PERMANENT MAXILLARY INCISOR TEETH

For the study of the anatomical site-distribution of disease, dental caries has some conspicuous advantages: it is a very

114

common condition and attacks are mainly confined to specific sites. Most mouths, especially those of young individuals, have many teeth – so giving abundant data – while the distinctive morphology of each tooth type provides a variety of evidence. The diagnosis of overt clinical dental caries is fairly straight-forward, and differences in judgment between independent examiners are small. Moreover, the evidence is quantitative and it is therefore susceptible to mathematical analysis. The only major disadvantage is the loss of teeth, but even this can be allowed for. Because the anatomical distribution of caries attacks cannot as yet be interpreted by the orthodox acidogenic theory of dental caries, this is a cogent reason for studying them (Jackson 1968; Jackson *et al.* 1967).

So much evidence, with so many ramifications is in fact forth-coming that we are confronted with an *embarras des richesses*. In this short chapter I have to be highly selective, but permanent maxillary incisor teeth exhibit the essential general features I wish to emphasise, and the detailed discussion will be confined to the distribution of carious lesions between pairs of selected sites in these teeth. The epidemiological data analysed by Jackson (1968) are summarised in Fig. 8.1.

ANATOMICAL PATTERNS IN RELATION TO AGE

A site on a tooth is considered to have suffered an attack of caries if a filling (F) is present, or if active caries (D, for decay) can be detected clinically. Every pair of sites considered in Fig. 8.1 shows one general feature: above the age of 20 to 30 years the ratio of single to double attacks in the population becomes effectively constant. Between 12 and 20 years this ratio can show a falling characteristic, as in (a) to (c); or near constancy, as in (d) and (e); or a rising characteristic, as in (f).

We also find, in any age group, that the prevalence of DF attacks on the right site (e.g. R Ce m, R Lat pit), is approxi-mately equal to the prevalence on the left homologous site (Jackson 1968; Jackson *et al.* 1967). In other words, right-left symmetry of attack is generally observed at homologous sites, considering the population as a whole. However, as Fig. 8.1 (e) and (f) imply, some individuals have a lesion on the right only,

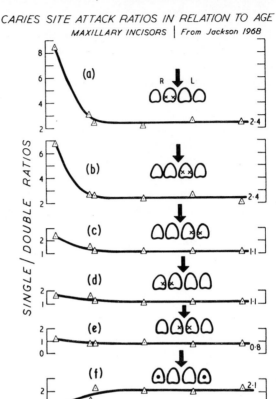

CARIES SITE ATTACK RATIOS IN RELATION TO AGE
MAXILLARY INCISORS | From Jackson 1968

Fig. 8.1　Caries attack ratios in the population, between pairs of sites on permanent maxillary incisors, in relation to age. Replotted from Jackson (1968). The point at 19 years refers to first year undergraduates at Leeds University, previously resident anywhere in the U.K.; the point at 20, and at other years, refers to local, mainly Leeds patients. (a) Single/double attack ratios for the mesial (m) and distal (d) surfaces of the right central (R Ce) maxillary incisor. A 'single attack' involves caries – a decayed (D), or filled (F), site – at the R Ce m *or* R Ce d surface; a 'double attack' involves caries (D or F) at both surfaces. The ratio stabilises at about 2·4 from 20 years and upwards. (b) Similar data for the left central maxillary incisor. Again, the ratio stabilises at about 2·4. (c) Single/double attack ratios for adjacent surfaces – left central distal (L Ce d), and left lateral mesial (L Lat m). The ratio stabilises at about 1·1, (d) Similar data for R Lat m and R Ce d surfaces. (e) Similar data for R Ce m and L Ce m adjacent surfaces. The single/double attack ratio stabilises at about 0·8. (f) Single/double attack ratios for R and L homologous sites – the lingual pits in lateral incisors. The ratio stabilises at about 2·1 above the age of 30 years.

some have a lesion on the left only, while others have lesions at both homologous sites.

But whether we consider homologous sites; sites on the same tooth, as in (a) and (b); or adjacent sites, as in (c), (d) and (e), one feature persists. Despite an increasing *prevalence* of attack with age (see Fig. 3.3), the anatomical *pattern* of site distribution remains effectively constant throughout adult life. The single/ double ratio 'freezes' at some fixed value which ranges from 0.8 to 2.4, depending on the particular pair of sites. Taking the example of central maxillary incisors: out of every nine adult individuals in whom both incisors are present, and in whom at least one Ce m carious lesion is present, 2 have a R Ce m lesion only, 2 have a L Ce m lesion only, and in the remaining 5, both R and L Ce m surfaces are carious. These ratios are maintained from 18 to over 50 years of age. They imply that certain sites, in certain teeth, in certain people, are completely resistant to dental caries.

PROBLEMS OF INTERPRETATION

Consider the anatomical distribution of caries which might be anticipated on the basis of the orthodox aetiological theory. This theory states that food (carbohydrate) débris is fermented by acidogenic bacteria, and that the resulting acid dissolves the surface enamel of the tooth to produce a carious lesion. Where adjacent surfaces such as R Ce m and L Ce m are concerned, the space between them is shared, and on the simplest view, we would expect that an attack on one surface would generally be accompanied by an attack on the opposite one. Hence, all attacks on adjacent surfaces ought to be double attacks, and the single/double ratio ought to be zero at all ages. Fig. 8.1. shows this prediction to be false. For all three adjacent surfaces – curves (c), (d), and (e) – the single/double ratio stabilises at about, or slightly below unity.

Unfortunately, it is difficult to modify the orthodox theory in a way that leads to quantitative prediction. Nevertheless, we could argue that the rate of progression of acid attack on the enamel is not exactly the same for adjacent surfaces and that local factors – of one form or another – are responsible for some discordance in attack. Discordance would be pronounced in

12-year-old children because at this age, cavities in more resistant areas might be absent or too small to be detected clinically. On this modified view, which postulates differential resistance, we should expect the ratios to change progressively with increasing age. Initially, only the susceptible areas would be attacked, but eventually the more resistant areas would succumb. Hence, the single/double ratio might be high initially but with increasing age it would be expected to fall progressively towards zero. This expectation is slightly closer to some of the observations than the first, because in curves (a) to (c) the single/double ratio falls appreciably between 12 and 20 years of age. However, the prediction remains fundamentally false because there is no further drop beyond 20 years of age, despite the increasing prevalence of caries with age. And in curve (f), the ratio actually *increases* between 12 and 30 years of age. We have little option, therefore, but to abandon these simple and modified versions of the orthodox acid theory.

Further modifications of the orthodox theory, involving random 'hits' (traumatic or otherwise) on the tooth enamel, in conjunction with an acid attack, have been tested and found wanting (Jackson *et al.* 1967). We have invited many defenders of the acidogenic theory to explain the observed single/ double ratios in conventional terms, but so far, neither they nor we have succeeded. A satisfactory explanation along conventional lines may be unattainable.

INTERPRETATION OF THE ANATOMICAL SITE SPECIFICITY OF
THE LESIONS OF AUTOAGGRESSIVE DISEASE

Mainly on the basis of age-distributions, we proposed that the *intrinsic* contribution to the multifactorial pathogenesis of dental caries is autoaggressive in character, and that odontoblasts probably constitute the target cells of the attack by the primary autoantibodies (Burch and Jackson 1966a). On this view, predisposition to caries – in any particular tooth, at any given site – is determined by genetic factors. The morphology of a given tooth is complex, and it follows from our theory of growth-control that the odontoblasts in specific regions of a given tooth, as well as those in different teeth, must have distinctive

TCFs. Mirror image differences between right and left teeth must derive from differences in 'right and left TCFs'. Whether or not a TCF is susceptible to attack by an appropriately mutant MCP is, according to theory, determined by the mutual *relationship* between these two macromolecules, and ultimately by the multiple genes that code for the MCP–TCF polypeptide chains. Consequently, some genotypes will have one set, or multiple sets of cells, at risk with respect to autoaggressive attack, and other genotypes will have no sets at risk. In other words, certain sites, in certain teeth, will be absolutely resistant to dental caries. Predisposition to dental caries generally, and to specific site-attacks in particular, will be determined by multiple genes coding for MCP–TCF growth-control molecules.

Consider the distribution of caries attacks between two specific sites S1 and S2, from the point of view of autoaggressive theory. To take a highly oversimplified example, suppose that a gene s has two alleles $s1$ and $s2$, and that the genotype $s1/s1$ is predisposed to caries at S1 but not S2; $s2/s2$ is predisposed to caries at S2 but not S1; and $s1/s2$ is predisposed to caries at both S1 and S2 sites. Assume the frequency of the $s1$ allele to be equal to that of the $s2$ allele $(= 0.5)$. Then from the Hardy-Weinberg law, the frequency of the $s1/s1$ genotype in the population will be 0.25 and equal to that of the $s2/s2$ genotype; the frequency of the $s1/s2$ heterozygote will be 0.5. Suppose that in each of the three genotypes, the disease process is initiated by a single random event, of the same average rate k, in each group. Also, suppose the average latent period between the initiation of the forbidden-clone and the appearance of caries is exactly the same in each of the three groups. It follows that, in the population as a whole, the age-prevalence (P_t, S_1) at age t, of S1 lesions only, will be exactly the same as that (P_t, S_2) of S2 lesions only, and that the age-prevalence $(P_t, S_1 . S_2)$ of S1 with S2 lesions will be exactly twice as high. Hence in this very simple example, the ratio of single attacks (S1 *or* S2) at a given age, to that of double attacks (S1 *and* S2) at the same age, will be unity at all ages. This prediction, based on highly simplified assumptions, is remarkably close to some of the observations. (See curves (c), (d) and (e) in Fig. 8.1.)

COMPLICATING FACTORS

According to the genetic scheme assumed above, everyone would be at risk with respect to caries at S1 and/or S2, but as we see from Fig. 3.3 only 60 per cent of all permanent maxillary incisors in the Leeds population are at risk with respect to caries, at one site or another. It follows that, in this population predisposition to dental caries at any specific site in maxillary incisor caries is polygenic. Furthermore, allelic frequencies may not always be 0·5, although the symmetry in the attacks between different pairs of sites (Jackson 1968; Jackson *et al.* 1967) suggests that some are. (By plotting the age-specific prevalence of site attack as a function of age, we can, of course, estimate the proportion of the population that is predisposed, to caries at that specific site, or combination of sites.)

Another complication concerns the lack of constancy of certain ratios in the 12 to 20 years age-range. In theory, this could arise in any one or more of the following ways: (i) the average rate of initiation of forbidden-clones (k) may not be exactly the same in $s1/s1$, $s2/s2$, and $s1/s2$ individuals; (ii) in one genotype, 1 clone may be required to initiate caries, but in another genotype, 2 or more clones may be required; (iii) where both sites (e.g. S1 and S2) are jointly at risk, the duration of the progression phase (latent period) may not be exactly identical at the two sites; (iv) the average latent periods may not be exactly the same in different genotypes .Given adequate age-prevalence data for lesions at specific sites, or combinations of sites, we can distinguish between these and other possibilities.

As in other autoaggressive diseases, various environmental factors may be expected to affect the duration of the progression phase. Epidemiological evidence shows that fluoride in the drinking water, at a concentration of about 1 part per million, prolongs this phase; acid producing bacteria may shorten it. Such agents may affect the rate of de-stabilization of dentine and enamel, once the integrity of the odontoblasts supporting the protein components of dentine and enamel has been destroyed by mutant MCPs.

Our theory predicts that a given site in a given tooth will either be susceptible to clinical dental caries or it will be absolutely resistant: this qualitative distinction is genetically determined. It is already well established that genetic factors are implicated in general caries susceptibility – see Finn's (1965) review – but so far, no large surveys of the inheritance of susceptibility to specific site attack have been published. However, from preliminary studies, my colleague Mr C. G. Fairpo is finding a higher concordance for caries site attack in monozygotic, than in dizygotic twins. The difference is highly significant ($P<0\cdot001$) and it confirms the genetic hypothesis.

Detailed analysis of the site-specificity of dental caries ought to illuminate some features of the 'tissue-code' and the genetic basis for right-left differences. The broad principles described here in connection with dental caries should also apply to the anatomical distribution of autoaggressive lesions in all complex tissues that are made up of different groups of cells, with distinctive TCFs.

CODA

To interpret the anatomical distribution of dental caries we are forced to go beyond the action of acid on enamel, and to consider the attack of mutant MCPs on complementary TCFs making up the plasma membrane of the odontoblast. We cannot deny, however, that the germ theory of disease, of which the orthodox aetiological view of dental caries is but a special example, has done more than any other theory to help alleviate suffering and to extend the average lifespan of man. On the other hand, the revolution inaugurated so brilliantly by Pasteur has probably done more than any other movement or concept to obscure the biological basis of disease. Yet over a century ago Virchow observed, with penetrating insight that, . . . 'pathology too must be referred back to the cell'. What more could a connoisseur of irony wish for?

9. THERAPEUTIC POSSIBILITIES. RELATIONS BETWEEN AUTOAGGRESSIVE DISEASE, CLASSICAL IMMUNITY, AND HYPERSENSITIVITY

'. . . I believe somatic mutation is a process of extreme importance in medicine . . . that cancer is a manifestation of the selective short-term survival of cells which have gained proliferative advantage by sequential mutation, and that old age and death represent the cumulative effect of a burden of somatic mutation in the body cells. Every one of these contentions has proved to be highly unpopular in both clinical and experimental circles.'

Sir Macfarlane Burnet, 1959

Doctors are concerned for their patients' welfare, and medical scientists aim strenuously to improve therapeutic and prophylactic measures. The very intensity of this zeal can, however, sometimes warp judgment, and doctors have been known to reject aetiological theories simply because no immediate prospect of prevention or cure is offered. Our analysis of the mechanisms of autoaggressive disease, cancer, and ageing does little to encourage a facile optimism – indeed a *Lancet* editorial (15 April 1967) has accused me of promulgating 'an Ibsen-like gloom' – but we must insist that the most important feature of a scientific theory, be it in physics or in medicine, is the extent of its truth or falsehood. And in the long run, a rational approach to therapy is likely to be better served by a true theory than a false one. I shall now discuss some therapeutic and prophylactic implications of our theory.

EUGENICS

In some autosomal dominant diseases, such as Huntington's chorea, the predisposing gene in question is of low frequency, and hence in principle its near-eradication would be possible if a thorough eugenics programme could be pursued. (New

mutations in the germ cell line will, of course, always reintro-
duce the gene.) But the difficulties in the way of eugenics – both
technical and moral – are severe. Firstly, if such schemes are
to be really effective, we must have tests to detect the predisposed person before symptoms of the disease appear.
The peak age at onset for Huntington's chorea is at 35 to 40
years, which is uncomfortably near to the upper end of the normal reproductive age-range. As yet, the young predisposed person
without the disease cannot be detected, although eventually biochemical and/or immunological analysis of MCP–TCF specificity should enable such people to be identified before puberty.
When this technical problem is solved it will remain for society
to decide what forms of persuasion, if any, should be applied
to encourage the carrier of the defective gene to refrain from
procreation. And, sooner or later, we shall have to decide
whether any form of compulsory sterilisation can ever be
justified. Scientific and medical knowledge has already forced
these moral and political questions upon us, and with our growing population, we can be sure their urgency will increase.

However, heterozygous fitness is commonly associated with
the alleles of genes predisposing to autoaggressive disease
(Chapter 7). When gene frequencies are high, and when the
homozygote, say $a1/a1$, is predisposed to a disabling disease, it
follows that the homozygote $a2/a2$ – where $a1$ and $a2$ are alleles
– will also be predisposed to a disabling condition, otherwise
the $a1$ allele would almost disappear from the population. (Of
course, a *very* high rate of mutation in germ cells, involving the
transition $a2 \rightarrow a1$, could also maintain a high frequency of the
allele $a1$; most geneticists would probably discount this
possibility.) Any reduction in the frequency of $a1$ attained by
eugenics would merely increase the frequency of $a2$. The
'$a1/a1$ disease' would be replaced by the '$a2/a2$ disease', and in
general, the frequency of the fitter heterozygote $a1/a2$ would
be reduced. (The proportion of heterozygotes for the a gene
in the population is at a maximum (one-half) when the frequency of the $a1$ allele is equal to that of the $a2$ allele, i.e.
when each is 0·5.) Thus, eugenics can only be clearly advan-
tageous when gene frequencies are already low.

Needless to say, when the entire population is predisposed to a
disease (and this is true, for example, of coronary artery disease),

eugenics has no scope; there is no 'good' gene pool to select from.

Although the average frequency of $a1/a2$ heterozygotes cannot be raised above the 50 per cent level by relying on natural reproduction and 'random' mating, this limitation could, in principle at least, be overcome by an artificial strategy. If vast banks of germ cells could be stored from $a1/a1$ donors of one sex, and from $a2/a2$ donors of the opposite sex; if fertilisation could be achieved; and if embryonic and foetal development could then be accomplished; then the outcome of this feat of technical virtuosity would be $a1/a2$ heterozygotes. So in theory, many common diseases such as inflammatory polyarthritis, diabetes mellitus, and schizophrenia could be eradicated from the population; popular acclaim for the means of eradication is more problematical.

Eventually, it will become possible to determine the phenotypic (immunological) specificity of foetal MCPs and TCFs, and hence we shall then be able to say that this foetus is predisposed to manic depressive psychosis, that foetus is predisposed to multiple sclerosis, and that one will be a victim of acute leukaemia during childhood. What use shall we make of such knowledge? Will this kind of evidence justify abortion? Who will make the decision? Will decisions based on such knowledge contribute to human happiness?

Consider the postulated random events – the spontaneous DNA strand-switching somatic mutations – that initiate the growth of forbidden-clones. Although the rate of this kind of mutation can be significantly *increased* in man (and other mammals) by substantial doses of ionizing radiation, there are no indications so far that mutation-rates can be significantly decreased under physiological conditions. When people can be safely despatched to the deep-freeze for prolonged cold storage, in a state of suspended animation, the *date* of onset of degenerative disease and ageing will be deferred, although the *effective* life-span will not be prolonged. Less heroic measures may be unavailing. But these are early days, and prophecy is unjustified.

NATURAL DEFENCE AGAINST THE FORBIDDEN-CLONE

We must now turn to the forbidden-clone itself. From the dependence of the average latent period on environmental factors, and from extensive clinical observations, we conclude that many factors influence the progress of the clone. As we saw in Chapter 4, the endogenous defence against forbidden-clones in one general class of autoaggressive disease is twice as efficient in XX females as in XY males. This is an important factor in the greater longevity of women. When we analyse mortality from heart disease involving coronary arteries (Fig. 4.10) we find that approximately 100 per cent of both men and women are at risk, and that rates of initiation are the same in the two sexes. But the average latent period in women (England and Wales, 1961) is about 20 years, in contrast to 10 years in men. Here, at least, the female is the stronger sex.

However, we must not place too much emphasis on the sex-differential in longevity. Swiss-Webster mice in a non-sterile environment show the usual sex-mortality pattern, with males being the poorer survivors, but when these mice are raised under germ-free conditions, the life-span in both sexes is greatly extended, and males then survive better than females (Gordon *et al.* 1966). Under sterile conditions, the female advantage in latent period is evidently offset by another sex-linked factor – most probably, the two-to-one (F/M) ratio in somatic mutation-rates at X-linked loci. In a non-sterile environment, these higher somatic mutation-rates will be more than offset by the greater relative importance of the latent period differential favouring females. Mortality from certain infectious diseases is also likely to be higher in male than in female animals of the same strain.

Precipitating and exacerbating factors in autoaggressive disease include drugs and many infective agents, and various other foreign antigens such as pollutants in the atmosphere, cigarette smoke, and the more specific factors such as allergens in connection with hay fever and other atopic diseases. Miller *et al.* (1967) report that smallpox vaccination and typhoid inoculation can precipitate and exacerbate attacks of multiple sclerosis. If more than one chronic autoaggressive disease is latent in a patient, and if these share defence resources, then an impairment of the common features of the defence will exacerbate these several latent diseases, more-or-less simultaneously. This phenomenon is often observed. For example, in patients with ulcerative colitis and episcleritis or iritis, eye lesions develop in association with attacks of colitis; furthermore, in one clinical series, every patient with iritis also suffered from simultaneous joint symptoms (Billson *et al.* 1967). Atwell *et al.* (1965) refer to a patient in whom an acute attack of psoriasis was always preceded by an exacerbation of Crohn's disease.

Mental stress is one of the most notorious allies of forbidden-clones and it has generated that extensive category: psycho-somatic disease. Disturbances along the celebrated axis: higher levels of the central nervous system, hypothalamus, pituitary, and adrenals, probably upset the balance between the endogenous defence, and the proliferating clone, through hormonal action. If longevity is your first objective, you would be well advised to become a country clergyman with an easy parish rather than an over-worked, city-dwelling, jet-travelling scientist. For those who have to live and work in cities, relief could be given to their overtaxed defence mechanism by eliminating atmospheric pollution, and infectious agents.

However, periodic diseases such as certain forms of manic depressive psychosis – in which the mood changes in a regular cycle from mania to depression – suggest that an undamped oscillatory interaction can occur between the intrinsic defence and the proliferating clone, without the intervention of extrinsic antigens. Many periodic disorders are known to be hereditary – see Reimann's (1962) review – and most, if not all, are probably autoaggressive in aetiology. Consequently, fluctuations in the levels of specific serum proteins and leucocytes should accompany the disease cycle. In a patient with periodic oedema, the only abnormalities detected during asymptomatic phases were a minimal eosinophilia and lymphocytosis, and a persistent abnormal gamma globulin (Clarkson *et al.* 1960). A marked neutrophilic leucocytosis occurred, however, during shock, and total plasma proteins rose abruptly from normal levels as the patient went into shock, to fall again during early recovery (Clarkson *et al.* 1960). Attacks and remissions in periodic diseases, if collated with the levels of specific plasma proteins and leucocytes, could reveal details of the endogenous defence against forbidden-clones.

At the opposite end of the clinical spectrum, disorders such as kuru (Burch 1968a), poliomyelitis (see Chapter 11), and hay fever (see below), appear to have an essential autoaggressive *component*, but symptoms and pathological complications result only when specific environmental factors intervene to aid the forbidden-clones. This interpretation accounts for the phenomenon of the 'carrier state', in which a person is infected with a micro-organism, but shows none of the usual complications of the disease process, such as the lesions of the central nervous system associated with poliomyelitis. It also accounts for (probable) genetic factors in connection with predisposition to kuru and poliomyelitis. We may therefore hope that other autoaggressive diseases, not at present known to be associated with specific viruses, mycoplasmas, bacteria, allergens, etc., will be found to manifest themselves only in specifically infected or invaded individuals.

I now discuss the nature of the endogenous defence mechanism which in some circumstances is so vulnerable to extrinsic agents. The following observations all corroborate the view that defence against forbidden-clones is mediated by immunoglobulins: (a) The incidence of autoaggressive disease is high in congenital and acquired hypogammaglobulinaemia. (b) Acute attacks of multiple sclerosis (Neumayer *et al.* 1956) are nearly always preceded by a *decrease* in the level of serum γ-globulin, while clinical recovery is accompanied by its restoration. My colleague De Dombal (1967b), finds that patients admitted to hospital suffering from a severe attack of ulcerative colitis always recover when their gamma globulin levels show a rising characteristic after admission; when, however, these levels are falling, the patient invariably has to proceed to surgery. (c) In systemic lupus erythematosus, the highest titres of immunoglobulin autoantibodies are found in patients with the mildest forms of the disease (Bielicky *et al.* 1966). (d) In one class of autoaggressive disease, the efficiency of defence is twice as high in females as in males. Beyond the age of 6 years, the overall level of IgM serum proteins is substantially and significantly higher in females than males (Butterworth *et al.* 1967). (e) Foreign antigens, introduced by infection, vaccination, and inoculation, often precipitate and exacerbate autoaggressive diseases presumably by competing for a common immune defence apparatus. (f) Plasmacytosis of the bone marrow is often observed in autoaggressive disease. (Plasma cells synthesise and secrete immunoglobulins.)

Contact between the mutant cell of the forbidden-clone and complementary normal cells will damage both (but especially the generally outnumbered forbidden-clone cells), and the release of autoantigenic débris will elicit a classical immune response directed mainly against the damaged, and therefore autoantigenic, cells of the forbidden-clone. Accordingly, the therapy of autoaggressive disease might benefit if we could elucidate the mechanism of defence.

THE CLASSICAL IMMUNE RESPONSE

Although many features of the classical immune response (acquired immunity) are well-established, they are difficult to interpret. So far, no comprehensive theory of acquired immunity has won general acceptance. The main intellectual task is to explain how the introduction of an antigen into an animal elicits the production of antibodies that combine specifically with the challenging antigen. The main therapeutic challenge is to discover how the efficiency of the immune defence against forbidden-clones can be enhanced.

Brienl and Haurowitz (1930) proposed that the antigen acts as a template for the formation of antibodies, but numerous experimental findings are inconsistent with this *instruction* theory, and it is now clear that antibodies are synthesised in the same way as many other proteins, such as enzymes, and haemoglobin chains (Nossal 1967). Burnet's (1957, 1959) clonal *selection* theory of acquired immunity has been briefly described in Chapter 2. It implies that potential antibody-producing cells in the immunologically-mature animal are committed cells, being capable of synthesising only one, or perhaps a few specific antibodies. Secondly, because of the postulate of random generation, through somatic mutation, of antibody patterns during embryogenesis, it is very difficult to avoid the conclusion that the specificity of response should be more-or-less independent of the genotype of the animal. Initial genetic differences should be largely or wholly obliterated by random mutation. Both these features of Burnet's theory are also implied by the more recent theories of Brenner and Milstein (1966), Smithies (1967), and Whitehouse (1967), but neither feature is supported by the extensive evidence from experimental immunology (Gorer and Schütze 1938; Scheibel 1943; Song and Sobey 1954; Sobey 1954; Arquilla and Finn 1963; Levine, Ojeda and Benacerraf 1963; Dineen 1964; Brand 1965; Gill 1965; McDevitt and Sela 1965; Pinchuk and Maurer 1965; Amkraut, Garvey and Campbell 1966; Feldman and Mekori 1966; Groth and Webster 1966; Sobey, Magrath and Reisner 1966; Vazquez and Makinodan 1966; Rose and Cinader 1967; Ripps and Hirschhorn 1967; Caron 1967; Benacerraf 1967; Ben-Efraim et al. 1967; Trentin et al. 1967). Furthermore, some recent theories (Brenner and Milstein 1966; Smithies 1967; Whitehouse 1967) of the origin of the variations in structure between one specific antibody and another, are at variance with current studies of the amino acid sequence of λ and κ (light) chains from immunoglobulins, myeloma proteins, and Bence Jones proteins (Hood et al. 1966; Putnam et al. 1967; Kabat 1967). However, the contribution (if any) of light chains to antibody specificity is not yet clear and until extensive amino acid sequence investigations of the variable portion of the Fd part of heavy chains are also available, the molecular and genetic bases of the structure of antibody combining sites will remain uncertain.

CLONAL INDUCTION THEORY OF ACQUIRED IMMUNITY

Our *clonal induction* theory (Burch and Burwell 1965) avoids the difficulties inherent in the classical 'instruction' and 'selection' theories. In our view, which is agreeably supported by the experimental evidence, variations in antibody structure are genetic in origin (see the above list of references), and they depend upon a very large number of distinctive genes being available to determine the specific amino acid sequences in the variable portions of the antibody combining sites.

Following Jerne (1955), we postulate that in the primary classical immune response: (1) the antigen first combines with preformed circulating 'natural' antibody. There is now excellent experimental support for this postulate (Kerman *et al.* 1967; see also Boyden's (1966) review). 'Natural' antibodies should be present, at low concentration, in the IgM 19S immunoglobulin serum protein fraction of the non-immunised animal. (It is possible, though not yet certain, that they are also present in the 7S IgG immunoglobulin fraction of maturing animals.) (2) Antigen (Ag) combines with specific complementary antibody (Ab) to modify the structure of the latter through an allosteric mechanism. (3) The changed configuration of the Ab macromolecule in the Ag . Ab complex, provides a signal to specialised reticular or macrophagic cells in lymph nodes and spleen, which thereupon ingest the Ag . Ab complex. (4) The complex is dissociated, and the retained Ag is digested, when possible, by enzymic action. Various authors have proposed that the antigen is 'processed' – i.e. structurally modified in some way – to induce antibody synthesis. In contrast, we have proposed: (5), the *antibody* is 'processed', and that in the primary immune response it is transferred from the reticular or macrophagic cells to initially uncommitted, multi-potential cells, of the antibody-synthesising series. We argue that, in these cells, many specific immunoglobulins, coded by many genes, are present in the cytoplasm, each at low concentration. (It seems likely that under *in vivo* conditions specific uncommitted cells are multi- but not toti-potential, they can synthesise some, but not all of the immunoglobulins the whole animal can produce. However, the experimental evidence concerning this issue is still inconclusive.) In Chapter 7 I showed that DNA strand-determination at MCP–TCF loci could be accomplished if the polypeptide chain product of the informational strand complexed with the non-informational strand, to block *m*RNA transcription from it. We have suggested that, in uncommitted cells of the antibody-synthesizing series, both strands of the DNA of a particular range of 'antibody specificity' genes are available for *m*RNA transcription, although each strand is *partially* repressed by the polypeptide product of the other. (6) When a particular processed antibody is presented to an uncommitted cell, it combines with the complementary anti-body (Ab_c) already present at low concentration. This further reduces the concentration of Ab_c available for DNA strand-repression, thus freeing the DNA strand for the synthesis of antibody (Ab) of the same specificity as the inducing, processed antibody.

REGULATION OF THE SYNTHESIS OF IMMUNOGLOBULINS

Our original scheme (Burch and Burwell 1965) made no provision for the homoeostatic regulation of the general level of immunoglobulin synthesis. Various observations (see, for example, Allansmith *et al.* 1967), point to a negative-feedback control. In its absence, successive antigenic challenges would produce successive increases in the overall concentration of circulating immunoglobulins. In health, however, these overall concentrations remain more-or-less constant throughout matur-ity although the concentrations of specific antibodies increase in response to many immunogenic episodes. Feedback regulation could be readily achieved if circulating immunoglobulins *uncombined* with antigens were recognised and phagocytosed by other sets of reticular and macrophagic cells. Processed immunoglobulins could then be transferred to lymphoid and plasma cells to inhibit immunoglobulin synthesis (see Fig. 9.1).

Two consequences of this regulatory scheme must be inter-polated. (1) An autoaggressive attack on one or more specific sets of macrophages processing Ab . Ag complexes, will block the classical antibody response to a distinctive range of antigens. Damaged macrophages will fail to transfer processed antibodies to immunoglobulin-, or antibody-synthesising cells. The extent of failure will depend upon the range of the committed, or pluripotential uncommitted, lymphoid or plasma cells associ-ated with the damaged macrophages. However, this deficiency will leave intact the general level of circulating immuno-globulins. A disorder answering to this description has just been reported by Blecher *et al.* (1968). (2) An autoaggressive attack on one or more specific sets of reticulo-endothelial cells processing uncombined immunoglobulins, will lead to over-

ANTIBODY SYNTHESIS : PROPOSED SCHEME

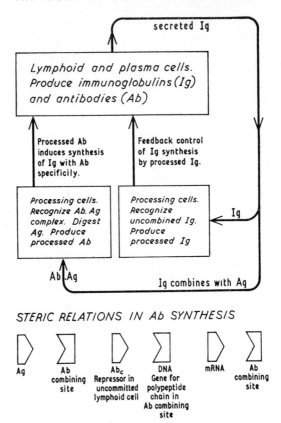

Fig. 9.1   Outline of scheme for antibody synthesis. The steric relations at the bottom of the figure should be compared with those proposed in connection with protein synthesis in Fig. 7.2.

production of one or more narrow ranges of immunoglobulins, as in Waldenström's macroglobulinaemia, the various forms of hypergammaglobulinaemia and multiple myeloma. Neoplastic plasma cells often synthesise homogeneous light (L) chains known as Bence Jones proteins. On the other hand, the heavy (H) chains of myeloma proteins are often heterogeneous (Poulik and Shuster 1964). These phenomena suggest that the specificity of a discrete set of plasma cells is characterised, in part at least, by a particular type of L chain. Consequently, the pluripotentiality of uncommitted cells synthesising immunoglobulins should depend upon the availability of multiple distinctive H chains. The Fd (variable) portion of the H chain is known to be involved in the antibody site which combines with antigen.

The average latent period in the lymphocytic class of auto-aggressive disease is twice as long in women as in men. Hence, X-linked genes may well code for polypeptide chains forming the 'variable' or specific section of the H chain in those immuno-globulins that provide for the endogenous defence against forbidden-clones of lymphocytes.

IMMUNOLOGICAL MEMORY

An animal generally produces an enhanced antibody response to a second or subsequent challenge from a specific antigen. This 'immunological memory' is mainly a property of the IgG class of antibodies. The phenomenon depends upon the persistence, over long periods of time (years in man), of cells specifically induced to synthesise antibody during the primary antigenic challenge. In the absence of circulating antigen, cells of the IgM series appear to revert fairly rapidly (over a period of days to a week or so) to the uncommitted state. Whether the IgG cell series is independent of the IgM series, or whether, as Nossal et al. (1964) suggested, IgG cells arise during the primary response from a change in the differentiation of dividing and committed IgM precursors, is still not clear (see, for example, Makinodan and Peterson 1966).

IMMUNOLOGICAL NON-RESPONSIVENESS

To repeat, in our *clonal induction* theory, the wide, but far from infinite range of antibody specificities present in a given animal depends primarily upon the large number of 'specificity' genes available for antibody synthesis, and *not* on a mechanism of somatic hypermutation during embryogenesis. Certain forms of immunological non-responsiveness can therefore be attributed to the absence from the genome of appropriate specificity genes.

The tolerance to certain self-proteins (such as insulin) circulating in the extra-cellular fluids could be of this form.

Non-responsiveness to circulating humoral MCPs and TCFs probably depends upon their general configuration. Phenomena such as steric hindrance could prevent antigenic determinants from gaining access to antibody combining sites. Normal TCFs on the outer surface of intact cells fail to elicit a classical immune response, because even when immunoglobulin 'natural' antibodies combine with them, the bulky complex fails to reach the specialised reticular or macrophagic cells in spleen or lymph nodes that process the Ag . Ab complex. In our theory, the transfer of processed antibody to immunoglobulin-synthesising cells, is essential to the normal immune response. It is well known, however, that if particular tissues from an animal are removed, homogenised, and then injected with adjuvant back into the animal, immunoglobulin tissue-specific autoantibodies are often elicited (Witebsky and Rose 1956; Rose and Witebsky 1956; Centeno et al. 1964). This evidence from experimental autoimmunity strongly supports the view that the normal state of tolerance between immunoglobulins and normal self-tissues depends upon the integrity of the tissues: the capacity to produce immunoglobulin autoantibodies is often present and it can be elicited by artificial procedures.

IMMUNOGLOBULIN AUTOANTIBODIES

Tissue-specific immunoglobulin autoantibodies are frequently found in many (but not all) patients with idiopathic 'auto-immune' (autoaggressive) disease. Previous chapters have excluded these immunoglobulin autoantibodies as the primary cause of the disease; Rowell and Beck (1967) have listed multiple reasons for making this rejection. Some immunoglobulin auto-antibodies reflect the response of the classical immune system to the antigenic débris released from the damaged target tissues. Mutant MCPs inflict the primary damage, although it can sometimes be intensified by tissue-specific immunoglobulin autoantibodies, as in autoimmune haemolytic anaemia where classical antibodies lyse erythrocytes.

It follows that cells bearing suitably mutant TCFs in target tissues will be damaged by normal MCPs and that the mutant, or not-self TCF débris, will elicit a classical immune response. Strand-switching mutation-rates of TCF genes in target cells are unknown: differences between growth-control and target cell nuclei in pH, ionic concentration, etc., might affect gene instability. If the rates of gene transitions in target and growth-control cells are at all comparable, mutant TCFs will abound, except during the early foetal stage. (Although the *proportion* of 'mutant' TCFs will be low at most, if not all ages, the total number of target cells in the adult human is $\sim 10^{14}$, and hence the *absolute number* of cells with 'mutant' TCFs will be large.) Consequently, immunoglobulin antibodies to many not-self TCFs will usually be present in the plasma because the interaction between normal MCPs and 'mutant' TCFs will yield the appropriate not-self antigens. Immunoglobulin auto-antibodies to normal TCFs will generally arise only when normal TCFs are damaged by mutant MCPs.

IMMUNOLOGICAL PARALYSIS

Massive doses of an antigen can induce a specific immunological paralysis to that antigen – a phenomenon we have attributed to straightforward mass-action principles (Burch and Burwell 1965). A very high concentration of antigen in the macrophagic cells processing Ag . Ab complexes will simply inhibit the dissociation of the complex:

$$Ag . Ab \rightleftharpoons Ag + Abp$$

so that processed antibody (Abp), is not made available to antibody-synthesising cells. Recently, another form of immunological paralysis to certain antigens has been discovered (Mitchison 1964), and this is produced by relatively low concentrations of antigen. This form of paralysis might result from an 'overshoot' of the negative-feedback control of immunoglobulin synthesis. More antibodies are produced than are necessary to neutralise antigen. Under certain critical conditions of antigenic dosage, the uncombined antibodies (immunoglobulins), after being processed, might drastically inhibit their own further synthesis.

THE FORBIDDEN-CLONE: THERAPY

Once an autoaggressive disease has started, we shall generally wish to restrain the proliferation of the forbidden-clone.

Obviously, the elimination of the mutant stem cell itself is an even more desirable objective. Complete and spontaneous remission of 'autoimmune' disease is sometimes observed. Occasionally, the mutant stem cell may either be eliminated by the defence mechanism, or it may undergo further mutation to a harmless form.

Because corticosteroid and A.C.T.H. therapy of 'auto-immune' disease is often successful, hormonal action may inhibit the rate of production of primary autoantibodies, and assist the defence mechanism. These benefits are perhaps greatest when the usual clinical course of the disease is charac-terised by a short, acute attack. To take the example of facial (Bell's) palsy, a substantial proportion (40 per cent) of attacks in untreated patients leads to irreversible denervation. However, if within 5 days of the onset of an acute attack, the patient is given a course of A.C.T.H. gel injections, complete denervation is nearly always prevented (Taverner *et al.* 1966; 1967). (I cannot refrain from mentioning that this treatment of facial palsy represents the first therapeutic success of our unified theory of growth and disease. My colleague Dr D. Taverner gave me the details of the sex and age-at-onset of his large series of patients with facial palsy. From their mathematical analysis (Fig. 4.22) I suggested that this disease has an auto-aggressive aetiology, and Dr Taverner decided to put the theory to therapeutic test. Therapeutic success in this instance prob-ably depends upon the ability of the drug to minimise the extent of the increase in concentration of the primary autoantibody during the initial attack. Above a certain critical level, the damage to the target tissue (? Schwann cells) becomes severe and irreversible; if the primary autoantibody concentration can be kept below this critical level, damage is transient and reversible.)

In many diseases, therapeutic advantage is more difficult to achieve. Certain glucocorticoids produce involution of lymphoid organs, delays in homograft rejection (involving MCPs), and they reduce immunological responsiveness to classical antigens (involving immunoglobulins). Hence the outcome of hormonal treatment of autoaggressive disease will depend upon the differential effects on mutant MCPs and defence immuno-globulins. In diseases with a progressive course, the chance of maintaining a suitable domination of defence over attack seems slender at present, but intensive investigation of the defence mechanism itself is clearly warranted, and it might prove rewarding.

If our theories of the classical immune response and the endogenous defence against forbidden-clones are valid, then the efficiency of defence should depend primarily upon the functional levels of two cell systems – the antibody-synthesising, and the antibody-processing cells. We need to determine the factor or factors which limit the capacity of the overall defence mechanism, and to find whether we can override or evade the natural limits by the use of artificial stratagems. If the chief bottleneck is the rate of synthesis of anti-forbidden-clone antibodies by lymphoid and plasma cells, then our therapeutic task would appear to be fairly straightforward. We need to produce anti-sera against forbidden-clones, and to inject these into the patient so as to maintain an adequate concentration of defence antibodies. Experience that is now being gained in connection with transplantation studies may prove to be invaluable in this context. Graft-rejection comes about when the (mainly) normal MCPs of the host – humoral and cellular – are complementary and pathogenic towards at least some of the TCFs of the graft cells. The anti-lymphocyte sera now being developed will be effective against the cellular MCPs of the host. I suspect that idiopathic kidney failure is often caused by autoaggressive disease, and hence it might eventually be easier, and more economical, to suppress the mutant MCPs of the host's forbidden-clone, than the normal MCPs that threaten the rejection of the kidney homograft.

If the major limitation of the endogenous defence system resides in the capacity of reticulo-endothelial cells to process antigen-antibody complexes, then our therapeutic task is likely to be severe. Mere addition of compatible macrophages, say, is rather unlikely to be effective, because the anatomical and functional relations between processing cells, and antibody-synthesising cells are evidently critical. The difficulty of inducing an immune response *in vitro* shows how demanding such conditions can be. Ways may be found to enhance the activity of the host's own processing cells, or to relieve them of a part of their burden. Fortunately, many investigations of the classical immune system are being currently pursued, and progress in this direction can be anticipated. Some recent investigations of immune suppressive drugs by Kimball *et al.* (1967) offer encouragement. These workers found no correlation betwen drugs which increased skin homograft survivals (and therefore depressed the host's MCPs), and those which suppressed humoral antibody formation. Drugs which inhibit forbidden-clones – and not normal MCPs or the endogenous defence mechanism – may therefore be discovered.

REMOVAL OF TARGET TISSUE

When the target tissue of the autoaggressive attack can be dispensed with, or replaced, then surgery can often be of immense benefit to the patient. The advantages of proctocolectomy in ulcerative colitis, when there is total involvement of the colon and rectum, are very real (de Dombal *et al.* 1966). However, the limitations of surgery are only too obvious. Many organs are indispensable, although much ingenuity has been displayed in finding substitutes.

SUBSTITUTIVE THERAPY. ORGAN TRANSPLANTATION

Occasionally, substitutive therapy can be practiced without the aid of surgery, as in the treatment of the responsive form of diabetes mellitus with insulin injections. Hormones, depleted by the autoaggressive attack on cells synthesising them, can therefore be supplemented artificially, at least in some circumstances. But currently, the most dramatic and newsworthy form of substitutive therapy is unquestionably organ transplantation.

By the careful selection of donor to minimise histoincompatibility between graft and host, and by the judicious suppression of the host's immune mechanism, it is hoped that long-term acceptance of not-self organs will be accomplished. I have the impression that the biological difficulties inherent in organ transplantation are sometimes underestimated, and that some of the more exuberant propaganda for spare-part surgery should be treated with reserve – except, perhaps, by the donors of research-grants. That the choice of a suitable donor of a kidney is less than straightforward is illustrated by the following statistics: out of twenty-seven cases where a kidney was transplanted from a monozygotic (identical) twin to the co-twin, only twenty recipients were alive one year after the operation, and in at least five cases, the transplanted kidney developed the original disease from which the patient suffered (Calne 1965).

Very frequently, autoaggressive disease is likely to be responsible for the original organ failure, and hence in such cases the transplantation of an organ with TCFs that are identical with the host's is doomed to failure: the host's forbidden-clone(s), unless restricted, must inevitably attack the transplanted organ. In this situation, we require grafts TCFs that are compatible *both* with the host's *normal* and *mutant* MCPs. For outbred populations, the graft selection problem is obviously severe, and for some combinations of normal and mutant host MCPs it might be insoluble. Suppression of the host's normal MCPs that are complementary to graft TCFs will be essential for the survival of partially incompatible grafts. Limits to survival might then be set by the rate of loss of cells from the graft. Under physiological conditions, stem cell loss from a tissue is made good through the symmetrical mitosis of viable stem cells, stimulated by MCPs. Selective suppression of the production of MCPs complementary to the graft would not help to replace cells lost from the graft. Non-selective suppression of MCPs would affect the replacement of cells in the host's normal tissues. But if our resources were adequate to curtail the production of specific MCPs, we should then be able to eradicate the host's forbidden-clone. And if that could be accomplished, the need for organ transplantation except, for example, in traumatic cases, might be obviated.

HYPERSENSITIVITY

It has long been known that people surviving certain infectious diseases rarely succumb a second time. The reason for this immunity is the persistence in the circulation of an adequate concentration of antibodies (mainly IgG) that are specific for the infective agent. When immunised, the neutralisation and elimination of the re-infecting micro-organisms is so rapid that symptoms of infection fail to develop.

At the beginning of this century, Portier and Richet (1902) discovered, however, that certain antigens do not induce a state of acquired immunity in certain animals. Instead, a first challenge produces a condition of sensitisation, and a second intravenous injection of the antigen produces a severe toxic reaction, which can even lead to death. This is *hypersensitivity*.

Two types of hypersensitivity reactions have since been delineated: *immediate* and *delayed*. Immediate hypersensitivity, or anaphylaxis, can be passively transferred from an affected to a recipient animal by means of serum, whereas intact living cells – probably lymphocytes – are required to transfer delayed hypersensitivity. Many observations support the widely-held thesis (Szenberg and Warner 1962; Archer *et al*. 1963; Isakovic *et al*. 1963; Miller 1963; Tyan and Cole 1964; 1967; Burch and Burwell 1965; Leskowitz 1967) that the part of the lymphoid system implicated in delayed hypersensitivity and in the homograft response, is based on a cell series separate from the one concerned with immunoglobulin synthesis.

We have proposed that immediate hypersensitivity involves the central humoral growth-control system, and that delayed hypersensitivity involves the cellular (lymphocytic) growth-control series (Burch 1968a; Burch and Burwell 1967). Immunoglobulins, and normal and mutant MCPs and TCFs, are all 'recognition' molecules, and they will combine with molecules that can gain access to, and are complementary with their binding sites. We must therefore consider the effect of 'hypersensitivity antigen' (HAg) combining with afferent humoral TCFs, on the feedback control of mitosis. If the resulting HAg . TCF complex is antigenic – as it is likely to be – it will combine with complementary immunoglobulin antibodies to elicit a classical immune response. TCFs bound in this way will be diverted from their normal processing cells in the growth-control system to the processing cells (e.g. macrophages) of the immunoglobulin system, and their afferent function will therefore be destroyed. After a primary challenge with HAg, there will be a small and transient increase in output of efferent MCPs. Provided the MCPs are normal, this will not be serious, and it should merely result in a transient hyperplasia of target cells. When the HAg antigen has been removed from the circulation, the return to normal should be rapid. However, a subsequent (secondary) challenge with HAg will lead to a swift removal of the HAg . TCF complex because now the animal is immunised to this antigenic complex and it has a relatively high concentration of IgG antibodies specific for this complex. This rapid reduction in the concentration of circulating TCFs will lead to a prompt increase in the ouput of MCPs related to the TCF bound to HAg. If any of these MCPs are suitably mutant, then serious acute damage to the target tissue could result. The accompanying anaphylactic shock may be due to the release of histamine from mast cells, which are the possible producers of certain humoral MCPs (Burch and Burwell 1965).

ATOPIC DISEASE. ALLERGY

Atopic diseases such as hay fever are often regarded as hyper-sensitivity conditions, and hence the above mechanism may well be involved in their pathogenesis. They can be viewed as

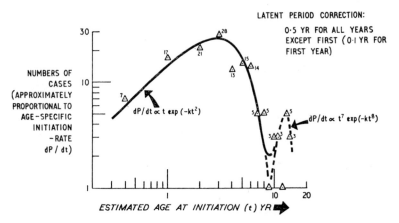

Fig. 9.2 Age-distribution of asthma (Richards *et al.* 1967). Numbers are small, but for onset before 15 years of age, two genetically-distinctive groups appear to be predisposed. For the early onset group, with a modal initiation age at about 2.9 years, $r = 2$ and $k \simeq 5.9 \times 10^{-2}$ yr^{-2}.

latent autoaggressive conditions that require a specific stimulus (given by HAg) for their expression. An allergen (pollen, etc.) is the equivalent of HAg, and its combination with TCF in the person with the appropriate dormant forbidden-clone, will initiate the sequence of events that leads to overt symptoms. Sex-specific and age-specific onset-rates for asthma, generally regarded as an atopic disease, give a satisfactory fit to 'auto-aggressive statistics' (Fig. 9.2). The precipitation of asthmatic attacks by mental stress should probably be attributed to its effects on the endogenous defence against the forbidden-clone.

10. CELLS, GROWTH AND DISEASE

'No cell lives by itself. It always depends on the environment which surrounds it, part of which is other cells.'

Paul Weiss, 1962

Evidence reviewed in Chapter 6 leaves little doubt that growth is centrally controlled. The cell systems responsible for this key function are less easy to identify, although they depend, directly or indirectly, on bone marrow; the executive cells, moreover, must be widely distributed throughout the body. Lymphocytes and basophilic granulocytes (including mast cells) are associated with many growth and disease processes, and the association may prove to be a causal one. Further evidence relating to this problem will be reviewed in this chapter. Associations between diseases; and between growth, morphology, and disease will also be described.

MALNUTRITION, GROWTH, AND AGEING

Normal body growth and regenerative growth are impaired by protein deficiency (Deo *et al.* 1967); even short periods of dietary inadequacy inhibit the local inflammatory response in rats (Taylor, P. E. *et al.* 1967). These phenomena, involving MCP production, are therefore very sensitive to starvation. In contrast, prolonged dietary deficiency is necessary to impair classical antibody production (Cannon 1949). Gill and Gershoff (1967) have found that total protein deficiency, severe enough to cause death from malnutrition, failed to affect the late secondary antibody response to a synthetic antigen. These several observations explain how starvation can extend the lifespan of mice and rats (McCay 1952). Evidently the rate of production of both normal and 'mutant' MCPs is reduced by an inadequate diet, whereas that of immunoglobulins – needed for defence against forbidden-clones – is barely affected. Consequently, the rate of proliferation of forbidden-clones is reduced, the severity of autoaggressive disease is diminished, and the lifespan is prolonged.

TEMPERATURE, GROWTH AND AGEING

Whereas starvation of mice and rats reduces growth but prolongs life, a lowered ambient temperature, just to complicate matters, increases both the growth and the lifespan of the annual fish *Cynolebias adloffi* (Liu and Walford 1966). In another fish *Carassius*, acceptance of homograft scale transplantation is greatly increased at 10°C, as compared with higher temperatures, up to 40°C (Hildemann 1957). This suggests that the intensity of the interactions between host MCPs and allogeneic graft TCFs increases with temperature. Hence the severity of the autoaggressive interaction between the host's 'mutant' MCPs and normal TCFs may also have a positive temperature coefficient. Such an effect will contribute to the increase in lifespan at low ambient temperatures. A reduction of the severity of the interactions between mutant MCPs, and complementary normal MCPs, will facilitate growth. Lowered temperatures will also, among other things, slow the rate of initiation of mutant MCPs (see Chapter 7).

LYMPHOCYTES; GROWTH OF TISSUE CULTURES; BODY GROWTH

Carrel (1922) emphasised the growth-promoting properties of various leucocytes in tissue culture preparations and in wound repair, and Humble *et al.* (1956) came to the conclusion that the lymphocyte . . . 'furthers the processes of growth and division of all cells regardless of their nature'. It is commonly held (see, e.g. Loutit 1962) that the lymphocyte has a trophic or nourishment function and this view is close to our own. Although the fate of the lymphocyte, once it has stimulated symmetrical mitosis *in vivo* is unknown, it must be either modified or destroyed to avoid confusion in the growth-control circuit. In tissue cultures, lymphocytes are often seen inside cells, and occasionally, the cells are in mitosis. This phenomenon was discovered by Humble *et al.* (1956) and they gave it the name 'emperipolesis', meaning 'inside round about wandering'.

Metcalf (1964) has demonstrated a remarkable parallelism

between the curves: (i) for the age-dependence of the rate of total thymic lymphocyte production in male C3H mice; and (ii) for the age-dependence of the weekly increase in body weight. He suggests, in complete conformity with our theory, that lymphocytes or their breakdown products might be concerned with the regulation of certain forms of mitosis in tissue cells.

Functionally, 'lymphocytes' are probably non-homogeneous. Clinically and experimentally, at least two populations of these cells can be distinguished (Peterson *et al.* 1965; Weber 1966; Clawson *et al.* 1967; Miller 1967; Craddock *et al.* 1967). One population, in which the cells are characterised by a small number of individual ribosomes in the cytoplasm and a short life, is likely to be concerned with growth-control. The other, in which the cells are long-lived and have numerous polyribosomes is probably associated with the synthesis of IgM immunoglobulins.

ALPHA-2 MACROGLOBULINS; GROWTH OF TISSUE CULTURES; BODY GROWTH

Healy and Parker (1966) have reviewed evidence for mitotic stimulation by the α_2-macroglobulin fraction in tissue cultures. A low molecular weight (40 000 to 50 000) α_1-acid glycoprotein also appears to be involved in growth promotion, at least in tissue cultures. The stimulation of symmetrical mitosis by humoral MCPs *in vivo* may, therefore, be a complex process involving the participation of co-factors. Alternatively, one class of α-globulin may normally stimulate symmetrical-, and the other, asymmetrical-mitosis.

From a study of the concentration of serum α_2-macroglobulin from healthy people as a function of sex and age Ganrot and Schersten (1967) conclude that this class of protein is involved in growth processes. The age-dependence of α_2-macroglobulin levels differs from that of immunoglobulins, and maximum concentrations of α_2M coincide with the adolescent growth-spurt.

Various physiological and pathological conditions produce an increase in the concentration of an α_2-macroglobulin, often called 'acute phase macroglobulin'. Hanna *et al.* (1967) concluded that the factors common to all conditions provoking this response are tissue injury, cell death, or both. The loss or death of tissue behind blood-tissue barriers, will, of course, stimulate the flow of humoral MCPs to effect tissue regeneration in an attempt to restore the *status quo*. Hanna *et al.* (1967) discovered that a 19S α-macroglobulin fraction increased survival among mice irradiated with a dose of 750 roentgens of X-rays. This α-macroglobulin also enhanced recovery of haematopoietic, including erythropoietic cells, in heavily irradiated mice.

BONE MARROW, GROWTH, AND ACUTE RADIATION DEATH

When most mammals, including species as disparate as mice and men receive large acute doses of ionizing radiation (some 500 rad of X- or γ-rays), about 50 per cent of the irradiated population die within 30 days. The main cause of acute radiation death at this dose level is a failure of the blood-forming organs.

Large acute doses of radiation destroy the proliferative capacity of a high proportion of cells. I have proposed that acute radiation death ensues when the proliferative capacity of every stem cell, in at least one central growth-control element that is essential to life, is destroyed by direct or indirect processes (Burch 1966c, 1967b). Target cells will also be killed by the radiation. If the central mitogenic stimulus is greatly diminished or eliminated, then regeneration and replacement of target cells will be grossly retarded or prevented.

Curves of the surviving fraction of animals (log-scale), against dose (linear-scale), when taken in conjunction with comparable curves for cell survival, enable us to make a crude estimate of the number of cells comprising a particular central growth-control element (Burch 1968c). I estimate this number to be of the order of 20, although it may of course differ from element to element. Assuming the number of growth-control stem cells in the bone marrow of man to be $\sim 2 \times 10^9$ (see Burch 1965) then, very roughly, the total number of growth-control elements will be $\sim 10^8$.

The central role of the bone marrow in acute radiation death is fully documented (see many papers and references in Annals N.Y. Acad. Sci., Vol. 114, Art. 1, 1964, and also Micklem *et al.*

1966). Shielding of only a small portion of the bone marrow – say one hind limb of a mouse – can prevent acute radiation death, and furthermore, normal bone marrow injections given after a dose of about 800 to 1000 rads often prevent this form of death. In Chapter 6, I referred to the restoration of liver regeneration in X-irradiated rats by bone marrow injections (Czeizel *et al.* 1962). The protection through parabiosis, against the lethal effects of large doses (1200 to 2400 R) of X-rays on rats is also of great interest (Carroll and Kimeldorf 1967). From this latter experiment we may conclude that factors circulate in the blood, and that they flow from the unirradiated parabiont to assist tissue regeneration (notably intestinal at these high dose levels) in the heavily-irradiated partner.

Full thickness excisions of skin evoke extensive symmetrical mitosis during the course of wound healing. The rate of healing of such lesions is greatly retarded in heavily-irradiated rats, and particularly in those animals subsequently succumbing to acute radiation death (Stromberg *et al.* 1967). When the hind limbs and pelvis are shielded from X-rays, an initial delay in wound healing is still seen (most peripheral MCPs will have been destroyed by the irradiation), but the subsequent rate of contracture of the wound, and its final appearance, are similar to those of unirradiated control animals (Stromberg *et al.* 1967).

BASOPHILS, MAST CELLS AND HUMORAL MCPs

So far as I am aware (in late 1967) no published observations bear directly on the nature of the cells synthesising humoral MCPs. Elsewhere, I have reviewed extensive evidence showing associations between tissue mast cells and the phenomena of growth, immediate hypersensitivity, and humoral auto-aggressive disease (Burch 1968a).

Some authors have believed that mast cell precursors are lymphocytes, but in view of the close morphological and bio-chemical parallels between mast cells and basophilic granulo-cytes, it is more attractive to regard the mast cell as the most mature member of the basophil series. Basophil counts are enormously raised in chronic myeloid leukaemia, and to a lesser extent in polycythemia vera and ulcerative colitis (Shelley and Parnes 1965; Sampson and Archer 1967). In Chapter 11, I follow other authors in arguing that the several forms of lymphocytic and myelogenous leukaemias are fundamentally auto-aggressive disorders. Grossly elevated levels of basophils in chronic myeloid leukaemia should therefore correspond to the proliferating forbidden-clone. The age-patterns of poly-cythemia vera (Burch 1966c), and ulcerative colitis (Fig. 4.21 a to g), suggest they are both autoaggressive disorders involving humoral (α_2-globulin) primary 'autoantibodies'. Serological studies of patients with ulcerative colitis strongly support this proposal (de Dombal 1967b).

Even more significant are the changes in basophil levels in immediate hypersensitivity. During sensitization to an antigen, the basophil count rises and it remains at an elevated level when sensitisation has occurred. If the patient is now challenged again with the antigen, a dramatic basopenia is often observed, resulting in anaphylaxis (Shelley and Parnes 1965). As we shall see in Chapter 11, our theory predicts this sequence of changes. I therefore arrive at the hypothesis that basophilic granulocytes and mast cells are components of the humoral system of growth-control. However, I am unable to exclude the possibility that tissue mast cells may help to regulate asymmetrical cell division.

From extensive dermatological studies, Asboe-Hansen (1964) arrived at analogous conclusions where mast cells are concerned 'Mast cells participate in innumerable disease processes of the skin, and skin pathology depends to a large extent on the activity of mast cells' . . .. 'The mast cell is in a key position in the processes of growth, regeneration and repair. It supplies the fundamental material that is needed for any growth to take place.'

LYMPHOID DEPLETION, THYMECTOMY, AND WASTING DISEASE

The general relation between lymphoid depletion, secondary disease, wasting, and runting, is very well known (Loutit 1962).

Recent experiments with antilymphocyte serum provide further confirmation (Denman and Frenkel 1967). Inbred rats were first made tolerant to rabbit IgG immunoglobulin. These tolerant animals were then injected daily with rabbit anti-rat-lymphocyte globulin, for periods of up to 1 month. Lymphocyte depletion and a form of wasting disease developed in the rats. From these and previous experiments, Denman and Frenkel (1967) conclude . . . 'that "wasting disease" results whenever the lymphoid mass is reduced below a critical level irrespective of the manner employed to produce this effect'.

Following the many pioneering observations of Grégoire, the rôle of the thymus has latterly attracted much attention. Neonatal thymectomy in several species is often followed by a wasting disease that is similar to runting (Parrott and East 1962; Miller 1962; Arnason *et al.* 1962; Sherman and Dameshek 1963). Wasting is prevented, however, if thymectomy is delayed until several days after birth, or if the neonatally thymectomised mouse is germ-free (McIntire *et al.* 1964). Conversely, wasting can be induced in neonatal (non-thymectomised) mice by injecting large doses of *sterile* bacterial vaccines (Ekstedt and Nishimura 1964). Thymectomy can also prolong the survival of allogeneic skin grafts for certain donor-host mouse strain combinations (Martinez *et al.* 1962).

The thymus, we suggest, serves as the first 'relay-station' in the lymphoid growth-control system (Burch and Burwell 1965), and there is little doubt (see Micklem *et al.* 1966, and Yoffey's 1966 review) that this organ is seeded by lymphoid cells from the bone marrow. Probably, growth-control lymphocytes are matured by the thymus (see Chapter 11), and the relative atrophy of the organ during adolescence and adult life (Boyd 1932) is consistent with this view. During regenerative and compensatory growth, and after heavy localised radiation of a part of the abdomen (Jansen *et al.* 1964), the thymus bulk is greatly reduced, suggesting that a heavy migration of cells occurs during repair and regrowth. Stressful situations have a similar effect on the thymus and they also exacerbate many autoaggressive diseases.

Neonatal thymectomy may well impair the growth and development of the endogenous defence mechanism directed against forbidden-clones proliferating in the bone marrow. By competing for finite defence resources, exogenous antigens such as viable micro-organisms, sterile vaccines, etc., facilitate the growth of forbidden-clones. Contact between cells of the forbidden-clone and their normal counterparts, results in mutual damage to both types of cell. Hence an impaired defence mechanism in the bone marrow not only enhances autoaggressive attacks, it also depresses growth. Wasting following neonatal thymectomy is likely to be a complex condition involving both autoaggressive disease and arrested growth. Thymectomy beyond the neonatal stage fails to produce wasting, because by then the development of the defence mechanism is, presumably, well advanced. Prolonged survivals of skin homografts suggest that the peripheral growth-control lymphocytes in the thymectomised mouse are not as robust as those in the normal animal. They have been deprived of the maturing action of the thymus.

RUNTING. GRAFT-VERSUS-HOST, AND HOST-VERSUS-GRAFT
REACTIONS

Medawar, Billingham, and Brent established that the injection of splenic or thymic cells from mice of certain inbred strains into newborn recipient animals of other inbred strains leads to runting. This condition shows atrophy of lymphoid tissue, loss of weight, diarrhoea, general debilitation, ruffled hair and failure to grow, followed by premature death. Runting, or transplantation disease, is attributed to a graft-versus-host reaction. On our theory, the active elements in the graft will be MCPs which have a complementary and pathogenic relation towards the MCPs and TCFs of the host animal.

Walford has exploited minor-grade histoincompatibility reactions between graft and host to support the 'autoimmune' (we prefer autoaggressive) theory of ageing which he pioneered (Walford 1962, 1967; Troup and Walford 1967). Tissue changes seen in allogeneic grafts, where the host's normal MCPs are complementary to the graft TCFs, should provide an excellent test of autoaggressive theories of disease. In general, graft changes will be more acute and more severe than those in spontaneous disease, because the variety and concentration of normal host MCPs under transplantation conditions will usually be higher than those of mutant MCPs in autoaggressive disease.

Burwell's (1963) original proposal concerning the role of the lymphoid system in growth-control sprang from his study of the reactions in lymph nodes to tissue transplantation.

The response of α_2-globulin plasma proteins to homografts has attracted less attention than that of lymphocytes, but the experimental findings are in remarkable harmony with our hypothesis. Several groups have found that the α_2-globulin concentration rises very soon after transplantation and before any increase in the β- and γ-globulin fractions can be detected (West et al. 1960; Peacock and Biggars 1962; Paronetto et al. 1965; Chiba et al. 1966). Alpha-2-globulin levels often rise continuously until the graft is rejected. After the graft is removed from the animal they return to control values, whereas the increase in γ-globulin tends to persist (Chiba et al. 1966). Apparently host MCPs, both humoral and cellular, first attack graft cells bearing complementary TCFs; the subsequent increase in immunoglobulin levels is induced by the release of particulate immunogenic fragments. The rapid increase in the concentration of host α_2-globulins (which should include humoral MCPs), parallels the rapid response in the immediate hypersensitivity reaction, which, I argued in Chapter 9, is mediated through 'mutant' humoral MCPs.

IMMUNOLOGICAL ENHANCEMENT

If a mouse is actively immunised with tissues from a donor animal bearing a tumour, or if it is passively immunised with hetero- or isoantisera, then the growth of a subsequent tumour graft from the donor to the host animal is facilitated. This is called *immunological enhancement*: the subject has been reviewed by Kaliss (1958, 1962). Similarly, rejection of non-neoplastic allogeneic skin grafts can be delayed in hyperimmunised mice (Kodama et al. 1967).

As postulated above, cellular destruction in allogeneic grafts is initiated by those humoral and cellular MCPs of the host that are complementary to graft TCFs. Wilson (1967) has shown that lymphocytes from rats actively immunised with allogeneic skin grafts can destroy cells of donor origin in tissue culture: 'Intimate contact between *intact* attacking lymphocytes and target cells appears to be mandatory for destruction to occur'. These destructive reactions take place in the absence of serum; neither the complement system, nor immunoglobulin antibodies are involved (Wilson 1967). During active immunisation with allogeneic tissues, the host's growth-control lymphocytes clashing with graft cells will sustain damage. Antigenic débris from these lymphocytes, as well as from graft cells, will therefore be released to elicit a classical immune response. The resulting antilymphocyte antibodies will reduce the numbers and the efficiency of host (MCP) lymphocytes complementary to graft TCFs. Antibodies can be expected to destroy damaged growth-control lymphocytes; undamaged lymphocytes and graft cells will be coated with a masking layer of antibodies which will protect the graft. In this way, the rate of destruction of neoplastic or normal allogeneic grafts by host MCPs is diminished. In other words, immunological enhancement is observed.

Related principles apply when an animal is challenged with a single type of foreign cell, such as xenogeneic red blood cells which can be lysed by 19S immunoglobulin antibodies. Initially, the growth-control lymphocytes of the host will interact with the foreign red blood cells; particulate antigens released from the red cells will then stimulate the production of 19S haemolysins. Mitchell and Miller (1968) have demonstrated the two-stage character of this sequence when mice are challenged with sheep erythrocytes. They found lymphocytes from the thymus or thoracic duct are required for the first stage, and a different type of cell, derived from the bone marrow, synthesises haemolysins.

Immunological enhancement and related phenomena support our general view of the relation between growth-control cells and the classical immune system. In particular, our interpretation of the defensive role of immunoglobulins in autoaggressive disease is strengthened. Mutant growth-control cells are first damaged by complementary normal growth-control cells, and the resulting particulate antigenic débris elicits the formation of immunoglobulin antibodies, some of which contribute to the endogenous defence apparatus.

CONNECTIONS BETWEEN GROWTH AND DISEASE IN MAN

The Swiss-type of hypogammaglobulinaemia in man shows lymphopenia, an undetectable or rudimentary thymus without lymphoid cells, *inexorable wasting*, absence of delayed hypersensitivity, and early death (Schaller *et al.* 1966; Fulginiti *et al.*

1966). These features are reminiscent of the effects of neonatal thymectomy in experimental animals, and the syndrome may therefore result from an ineffective *central* endogenous defence against forbidden-clones. An autoaggressive attack on the thymus, or a developmental failure of that organ might be responsible. The Bruton, sex-linked congenital form of hypogammaglobulinaemia shows no lymphopenia and no wasting. Probably, central defence against forbidden-clones in the bone marrow is largely or wholly intact, while the low levels of circulating gamma globulin result from the virtual absence of certain lymphoid and plasma cells from the spleen and lymph nodes.

Progeria provides one of the most conspicuous examples of the interrelations between growth, disease, and ageing (Walford 1962; Comfort 1963). A high incidence of 'autoimmune' disease, and a conspicuously enlarged and hyperplastic thymus (containing proliferating forbidden-clones?) is found in this condition of stunted growth and premature ageing (Gabr *et al.* 1960).

Werner's syndrome bears some resemblance to progeria, although it is not usually diagnosed before 20 years of age. It is characterised by a failure of growth, a senile appearance involving the early greying and loss of hair, premature skin changes, cataracts, a tendency to diabetes, osteoporosis, vascular disorders, early menopause, and death usually before 50 years of age. The mean height of men suffering from the syndrome is only 5 ft. 1 in., and of women 4 ft. 9½ in. (Epstein *et al.* 1966). This syndrome is believed to be inherited as an autosomal recessive. A pleiotropic gene evidently predisposes to autoaggressive disease of several tissues (including hair follicles, eye lens, pancreas, and bone) which lie behind blood-tissue barriers. The age-distributions of the various diseases affecting these tissues (Epstein *et al.* 1966) indicate a high rate of somatic mutation, probably of the pleiotropic predisposing gene. Production of mutant MCPs – which will interact with complementary normal MCPs – will lead to a failure of growth. Interestingly, the thyroid is generally normal, the pituitary shows no signs of dysfunction, and growth hormone has not been found to be abnormal or deficient either in this syndrome or in progeria.

CONGENITAL ABNORMALITIES

Formation of one or more mutant MCPs during embryo-genesis may result in the early failure of one or more growth-control elements, and the appearance of congenital abnormali-ties at birth. Some abortions and still-births may have a similar pathogenesis. Because the mutation of MCP genes is a random process, monozygotic twins may or may not be concordant for developmental abnormalities, depending on the chance that similar events occur in both twins, at comparable stages of development. Discordance is often observed between mono-zygotic twins for unilateral pulmonary agenesis (Booth and Berry 1967), and it can be readily explained in this way. Combining all reported studies of congenital heart disease where diagnoses were precise, Nora *et al.* (1967) found that 25 per cent of monozygotic and 4·9 per cent of dizygotic twins were concordant for congenital heart disease. A concordance ratio of about 5 to 1 between the two types of twins suggests that predisposition to congenital heart disease is polygenic, and that 2 loci might be implicated (see Burch 1964b,c).

MUTANT MCPs AND HYPERPLASIA

That certain mutant MCPs may promote excessive mitosis (hyperplasia) in the target tissue bearing complementary TCFs, is seen vividly in the 'enormous active growth of the epidermis' (Shelley and Arthur 1958) in psoriatic lesions. Another example is found in pannus formation in the synovium of arthritic joints, and yet another is provided by the thickening of the intimal lining of ageing arteries. A common cause of failure of transplanted kidneys in man is, significantly enough, an obliterative vascular change, which has been attributed to host-versus-graft immune attack (Porter *et al.* 1963).

Chapter 11 describes examples of more complicated relations between autoaggressive and proliferative disorders.

MORPHOLOGY AND DISEASE. POSITIVE AND NEGATIVE ASSOCIATIONS

Of the many associations between morphology and disease, one is so obvious we can easily overlook it – the differences in the spectrum of diseases in men and women. The several sources of these complex sex-differences in autoaggressive disease were described in Chapter 4. Inevitably, they derive in a rather direct way, from genes on the X and/or Y chromosomes.

Alter (1966) has reviewed the fascinating connections between finger-print patterns (dermatoglyphics) and disease. Both autosomal and sex chromosomal *aneuploidy* (an abnormal *number* of autosomal or sex chromosomes) together with gross chromosomal *aberrations* (translocations and deletions) give rise to abnormal dermatoglyphics. However, few theories of disease predict that a number of single gene disorders (including Huntington's chorea), together with polygenic disorders such as schizophrenia and psoriasis, might be accompanied by unusual finger-print patterns. They are, and they can be explained by our thesis that numerous genetically-based age-dependent diseases (such as those mentioned) arise from somatic mutations in cells of the central growth-control system. Because many different tissues share common histocompatibility antigens, certain genes must code for polypeptide chains in many MCP–TCF elements. Hence, if such a gene, or a combination of genes predisposes to a given autoaggressive disease, then that disease will be associated with certain morphological features of many MCP–TCF elements.

Various diseases will be positively associated – in the same patient, and/or in a given family – when predisposing genes, or gene-combinations, code for polypeptide chains in more than one MCP–TCF element. Equally, if alleles $a1/a1$ in homozygous combination predispose to disease D1, and the alternative alleles $a2/a2$ at the same autosomal locus predispose to disease D2, then D1 and D2 will never arise in combination. Cobb and Hall (1965) claim rheumatoid arthritis to be positively associated with tuberculosis and peptic ulcer, while this group of diseases is negatively associated with myocardial infarction, obesity and hypertension. Perhaps the best known example of positive association is between autoaggressive diseases of the adrenals (Addison's disease), the thyroid (Hashimoto's thyroiditis), gastric parietal cells (pernicious anaemia), and the pancreas (diabetes mellitus) – see, for example, Irvine *et al.* (1965). Logically, there must be negative associations between specific morphological characters and certain autoaggressive diseases.

Although much of the evidence discussed in this chapter can be interpreted in several ways, the bizarre associations between fingerprint patterns and disease are not explained by most aetiological theories. Such associations follow readily from the postulate that many diseases result from somatic mutations in growth-control stem cells.

11. LEUKAEMIA, CHROMOSOMAL ABERRATIONS, BURKITT'S LYMPHOMA, HODGKIN'S DISEASE AND VIRAL DISEASES

> '*Autoimmunity and certain forms of leukaemia, notably of the lymphocytic variety, are fundamentally either the same disease or different expressions of the same disturbance.*'
>
> William Dameshek, 1965

Many authors have commented on associations, either in the same patient, or in the same family, between lymphocytic leukaemia, lymphosarcoma, acquired hypogammaglobulinaemia, other immunological deficiency states, and 'autoimmune' disease (Dameshek and Schwartz 1959; Kaplan and Smithers 1959; Green *et al.* 1966; Dameshek 1966, 1967; Fudenberg 1966; Miller 1967; Oleinick 1967; Smithers 1967; Peterson *et al.* 1967; Twomey *et al.* 1967). Dameshek's opinions are shared by Peterson *et al.* (1967): 'The association of hypogammaglobulinaemia [Bruton's X-linked congenital form], lymphocytic malignancies and autoimmune diseases in this genetically determined syndrome supports the postulate of a common basic pathogenesis for all three phenomena.'

Connections have also been found between myeloproliferative disorders – mainly chronic myeloid leukaemia and Di Guglielmo's syndrome on the one hand – and on the other, hypergammaglobulinaemia (sometimes associated with the production of relatively homogeneous immunoglobulins), lymphosarcoma, reticulum cell sarcoma, and immunoglobulin autoantibodies (Joseph *et al.* 1966; Finkel *et al.* 1966; Ritzmann *et al.* 1966).

Burnet (1965) describes a forbidden-clone as a 'conditioned malignancy'. Where then do we draw the dividing lines – if any – between the growth of a forbidden-clone, myeloproliferative and lymphoproliferative disorders, and chronic and acute leukaemias?

In this chapter I shall follow other authors in suggesting that leukaemia, Burkitt's lymphoma, and Hodgkin's disease are all autoaggressive ('autoimmune') disorders. However, the arguments I shall deploy are new, and they help to reinforce the earlier proposals. The identity of the target tissue in these autoaggressive diseases is of special importance to our unified theory of growth and disease. Furthermore, the age-distribution of childhood leukaemia in patients with Down's syndrome, most of whom have three chromosomes 21 instead of the normal two, powerfully supports the view that the random initiating events in autoaggressive disease are a form of somatic gene mutation.

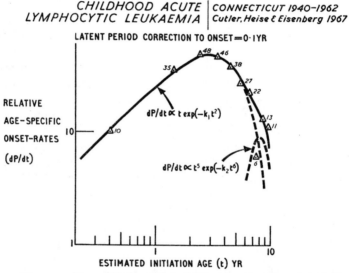

Fig. 11.1   Data of Cutler *et al.* (1967) for acute lymphocytic leukaemia in childhood; Connecticut 1940 to 1962. Sexes combined. For the early onset-group, $r = 2$; $k_1 \simeq 5.6 \times 10^{-2}$ yr^{-2}; for the late onset-group $r = 6$; $k_2 \simeq 3.2 \times 10^{-6}$ yr^{-6}. Latent period correction (initiation to *onset*) is 0.1 yr.

AGE DISTRIBUTIONS OF CHILDHOOD LEUKAEMIA

If a disease is autoaggressive in aetiology, then according to my general theory, its sex- and age-specific initiation-rates should conform to the model statistics described in Chapter 4. (The converse, of course, does not necessarily follow.) Age-distributions of acute leukaemia in childhood both in the sub-population of Down's syndrome (mongoloid) patients, and in the general non-mongoloid population, are illustrated in Figs 11.1 to 11.3.

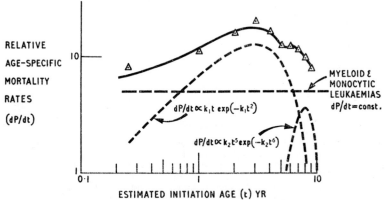

CHILDHOOD LEUKAEMIA | *OXFORD SURVEY*
SEXES COMBINED | *Lashof & Stewart 1965*

1796 non–mongoloid deaths: ENGLAND & WALES 1953–1960

LATENT PERIOD CORRECTION=0·5YR (0·25YR for first year of life)

Fig. 11.2 Data of Lashof and Stewart (1965) for all forms of leukaemia in childhood; England and Wales, 1953 to 1960. Sexes combined. Mortality-rates for acute myeloid and monocytic leukaemias are almost age-independent: that is, $dP/dt \simeq$ constant. Values of k_1 and k_2 are the same as for Fig. 11.1. Latent period correction (initiation to *death*) is 0·5 year, (0·25 year for the first year of life).

The four main diagnostic categories in childhood acute leukaemia are lymphatic, myeloid, monocytic, and unspecified. In non-mongoloids, the age-specific mortality-rates of acute myeloid and monocytic leukaemias are almost independent of age, but lymphatic leukaemias generally show a peak in mortality at 3 to 4 years of age (Lashof and Stewart 1965; Stewart 1967; Cutler *et al.* 1967; Fraumeni and Miller 1967). In mongoloids, the age-distribution of myeloid and monocytic leukaemias (Stewart 1967) does not differ significantly from that of lymphatic leukaemias, but when broken down in this way, the numbers are too small for definitive analysis. Although more non-mongoloid boys are affected by childhood leukaemia (all types) than girls, the shape of the age-distribution and the

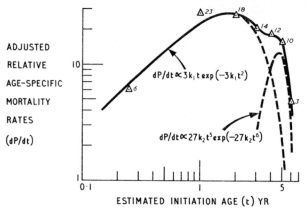

CHILDHOOD LEUKAEMIA | OXFORD SURVEY
SEXES COMBINED | Lashof & Stewart 1965

86 mongoloid deaths : ENGLAND & WALES 1943–1964

LATENT PERIOD CORRECTION=0·5YR(0·25YR for first year of life)

ADJUSTED RELATIVE AGE-SPECIFIC MORTALITY RATES (dP/dt)

$dP/dt \propto 3k_1 t \exp(-3k_1 t^2)$

$dP/dt \propto 27k_2 t^5 \exp(-27k_2 t^6)$

ESTIMATED INITIATION AGE (t) YR

Fig. 11.3   Data of Lashof and Stewart (1965) for 86 mongoloid deaths from childhood leukaemia in England and Wales, 1943 to 1964. The value of k for the early onset group is three times the value in Figs 11.1 and 11.2 ($3k_1$); for the late onset group it is 27 times that in Figs 11.1 and 11.2 ($27k_2$). Latent period corrections are the same as in Fig. 11.2.

position of the mode are the same for both sexes; accordingly, the data for both sexes have been combined. By making a latent period correction of 0·5 year between initiation and death (for all years except the first year), the data for non-mongoloids can be accurately represented by the sum of three initiation curves: (1) For myeloid and monocytic leukaemias,

$$dP/dt = k S \exp(-kt) \qquad [11.1]$$

(The factor $\exp(-kt)$ in this equation remains approximately unity so long as kt is much less than unity. dP/dt appears to be more-or-less constant up to $t = 10$ years, at least.) (2) For early-onset lymphatic and unspecified leukaemias, giving an initiation peak at 3 years of age:

$$dP/dt = 2k_1 S_1 t \exp(-k_1 t^2) \qquad [11.2]$$

(3) For late-onset lymphatic and unspecified leukaemias, giving an initiation peak at 8 years of age:

$$dP/dt = 6k_2 S_2 t^5 \exp(-k_2 t^6) \qquad [11.3]$$

A latent period correction of 0·5 year is also applied to the mortality data for mongoloids for all years except the first. The resulting age-specific initiation-rates are represented by the sum of two initiation-curves of forms identical with [11.2] and [11.3], except that the numerical values of the constants k_1, k_2, S_1 and S_2 are different. I find the value of k_1 in mongoloids to be three times higher than in non-mongoloids, changing the peak age of initiation for early-onset cases from 3 years to about 1·7 years of age. For late-onset cases, the value of k_2 is 27 times higher in mongoloids than in non-mongoloids, reducing the peak age of initiation for this group from 8 years to about 4·6 years of age. No indication is given of a significant contribution to the mongoloid data from an equation of the form of [11.1].

Absolute values of dP/dt are not quoted by Lashof and Stewart (1965), but the relative risk of leukaemia mortality in childhood is some 20 to 30 times higher in mongoloids than in non-mongoloids. Values of S_1 and S_2 for the mongoloid population are therefore much higher than the corresponding values S_1 and S_2 for the non-mongoloid population.

LEUKAEMIA: AETIOLOGICAL INTERPRETATION

Figures 11.1 to 11.3 show therefore that the initiation of childhood leukaemia, both in mongoloids and non-mongoloids, is described with satisfactory accuracy by 'autoaggressive statistics'. Early-onset cases with peak initiation at 3 years (non-mongoloids), and 1·7 years (mongoloids), both require two 'dependent-type' random events – most probably two somatic mutations in one cell – but the k value for mongoloids is three times that for non-mongoloids. For late-onset cases with peak initiation at 8 years (non-mongoloids), and 4·6 years (mongoloids), the number of 'dependent-type' initiating somatic mutations is 6 for both groups, but the k value for mongoloids is 27 times the value for non-mongoloids.

These differences in k values, associated with distinctive karyotypes, are of exceptional importance. They parallel the finding for diseases in which the k value in XX females is double the corresponding k value in XY males. I attribute this sex-difference to X-linked somatic mutations.

The 3 to 1 ratio in k values (mongoloids/non-mongoloids) is readily explained if the two events initiating early onset leukaemia affect homologous genes at a locus on chromosome 21 (Burch 1968a). The average rate (m_1) of the first event will be 3/2 times higher in trisomic mongoloids than in disomic non-mongoloids. When the first event has occurred, 2 genes remain at mutational risk in mongoloids, and only 1 in non-mongoloids. Hence, the average rate (m_2) of the second event will be twice as high in mongoloids. Consequently the k value (Lm_1m_2), will be three times higher in mongoloids than in non-mongoloids – in agreement with observation.

If the 6 'dependent-type' events initiating the late-onset form of childhood leukaemia correspond to the somatic mutation of two homologous genes, at each of three loci on chromosome 21, it follows from the above argument that the k value for mongoloids will be $3 \times 3 \times 3 = 27$ times higher in non-mongoloids. Lashof and Stewart's (1965) data are also in remarkable agreement with this prediction.

These kinetic relations between initiating events in mongoloids and non-mongoloids pose genetic issues similar to those raised by the commonly observed 2 to 1 (F/M) sex-difference in k values (see Chapter 7). At least two hypotheses can be considered. (1) The early-onset form of acute leukaemia arises only in children who have inherited the same kind of allele at a predisposing locus on both chromosomes 21 (non-mongoloids), or all three chromosomes 21 (mongoloids). The later-onset form of childhood leukaemia requires an analogous form of inheritance at three predisposing loci on chromosome 21. (2) Genes at these loci on chromosome 21 may be inherited in heterozygous arrangement, but, as with MCP–TCF genes on the X-chromosome, a directed DNA strand-switching 'mutation' occurs during embryonic induction to give precursor growth-control cells that are phenotypically homozygous. To help distinguish between these and other possibilities it will be useful to elucidate the obviously complicated genetics of childhood leukaemia.

The available evidence strongly supports the following postulates: (i) stochastic equations such as [11.1] to [11.3], and the more general equations of Chapter 4, describe the statistics of spontaneous gene mutations occurring in a cell population that is constant in number (L) from around birth to death; (ii) when Weibull renewal statistics are obeyed (general equations [4.4] and [4.5]; and particular equations [11.2] and [11.3]) the value of r often describes the number of gene mutations occurring in a single cell, out of L cells at mutational risk; (iii) acute leukaemia in childhood is fundamentally an autoaggressive disorder; (iv) early-onset lymphocytic leukaemia (mode at 3 years in non-mongoloids) is initiated by the mutation in a growth-control stem cell of both homologous genes at a locus on chromosome 21; and (v) late-onset childhood lymphocytic leukaemia (mode at 8 years in non-mongoloids) is initiated by the mutation in a growth-control stem cell of both homologous genes at each of 3 loci on chromosome 21.

The age-patterns of other diseases in mongoloids, and of diseases in groups with other chromosomal abnormalities, will be of great interest. Such studies will allow particular MCP–TCF genes to be assigned to particular chromosomes.

If a leukaemia is indeed an autoaggressive disease, the nature of the forbidden-clone itself – and that of the target tissue – are of outstanding theoretical interest. Before discussing these issues, I shall first consider some further associations between chromosomal abnormalities, autoaggressive disorders, and dizygotic twinning. I shall then go on to analyse the sex- and age-distributions of two other lymphoproliferative disorders, and of three viral diseases. Finally, I return to the biological implications of this varied evidence.

ORIGIN OF CHROMOSOMAL ABNORMALITIES

From 1963 onwards, numerous reports have appeared of positive associations between chromosomal anomalies, and autoaggressive disease in the affected patient, parents, and close relatives. Some of this bulky literature has been reviewed by Thompson (1965) in an article with 350 references.

A high prevalence of diabetes mellitus and thyroiditis has been found in patients with congenitally defective or absent ovaries (Forbes and Engel 1963; Engel and Forbes 1965). Only sixteen of their forty-eight patients with gonadal dysgenesis had the 'classical' XO sex-chromosome complement, and none of these XO patients had diabetes; eight of the remaining thirty-two patients (with X/isochromosome X, or mosaic sex chromosome anomalies, or no detectable cytogenetic abnormality), had diabetes (Engel and Forbes 1965). (An isochromosome X is believed to consist of two long arms from an X chromosome,

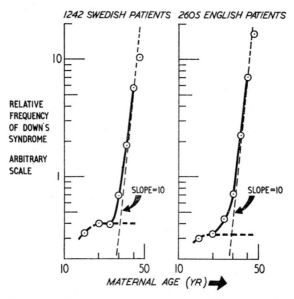

Fig. 11.4 Frequency of Down's syndrome compared with cytogenetically normal births (arbitrary scale), as a function of maternal age (Akesson and Forssman, 1966 – the statistics for 2,605 English patients were supplied to these authors by Professor L. S. Penrose). At least two groups of women are predisposed to producing offspring with Down's syndrome. The early onset group is relatively more prevalent, and the late onset group slightly less prevalent in the Swedish, as compared with the English population. About ten random events (somatic mutations) are probably needed to initiate the late onset form of this disorder. The relative incidence of early onset cases is probably effectively constant from the age of 20 years to the menopause. Given the existence of the forbidden-clone or clones causing 'germ cell disease' in the mother, we cannot, from these statistics alone, estimate the probability of chromosomal non-disjunction at a specific meiotic division.

instead of the normal one long and one short arm.) Thyroiditis was found in six of the forty-eight patients, whose average age was 42 years. Sparkes and Motulsky (1963) reported two instances, and Grumbach and Morishima (1964) one, of Hashimoto's thyroiditis in patients with an isochromosome X. Nielsen (1966a) discovered a high incidence of diabetes in the parents and close relatives of patients with Klinefelter's (XXY) syndrome; other investigators have confirmed these findings. Mellon *et al.* (1963) observed a high incidence of thyroid disease and thyroid autoantibodies in the mothers of children with Down's syndrome.

Because a high proportion of the antecedents of patients with gonadal dysgenesis had diabetes or thyroiditis, Forbes and Engel suggested that chromosomal non-disjunction occurs relatively frequently in families with a genetic predisposition to 'autoimmunity'. Fialkow (1964) elaborated this idea.

According to our theory, the growth of the germ cell series (which occurs prenatally in females) is under central control. It follows that, in the appropriate male or female genotypes, germ cells will become the targets of autoaggressive attack. Our suspicion (Burch *et al.* 1964) that chromosomal non-disjunction leading to Down's syndrome might often be caused by an auto-aggressive attack on germ cells, was first aroused by the importance of maternal age. Fig. 11.4 illustrates the relative probability of Down's syndrome births as a function of maternal age: the ordinate is proportional to the age-prevalence of women producing mongoloid offspring.

About ten random events are apparently needed to initiate the condition responsible for most mongoloid births beyond the maternal age of 30 years. Presumably a forbidden-clone is initiated and it leads to non-disjunction of chromosome 21 (or 22 ?) at meiosis. A bivalent or polyvalent autoantibody may penetrate to the cell nucleus to combine with complementary antigenic determinants present on homologous chromosomes. Through this specific binding, non-disjunction of chromosomes at meiosis would be prevented. Antigens with TCF specificity may therefore be associated with the nucleoproteins of chromosomes such as 21, X and Y, which feature relatively commonly in non-disjunction. (The occurrence of specific translocations between dissimilar chromosomes suggests that proteins with common antigenic – TCF – specificities may occur on more than one type of chromosome.) It follows that offspring inheriting abnormal complements of chromosomes must also inherit genes from the parent predisposed to autoaggressive disease of germ cells. Evidently, autoaggressive diseases of germ cells are positively associated in the parent with other autoaggressive disorders, including those affecting the thyroid and pancreas.

Nielsen (1966b) directed attention to another fascinating and related phenomenon: the association in the same sibship between Klinefelter's syndrome and dizygotic twinning. Following earlier indications, he found six pairs of twins in the sibships of eighteen patients with Klinefelter's syndrome. This frequency of twinning is some 3·4 times the 'expected' value, based on statistics for the general population.

DIZYGOTIC TWINNING

Dizygotic twinning results from the release and fertilisation of two oocytes at ovulation. An interference with the normal mechanism of oocyte release is therefore implicated. If this interference is produced by autoaggressive action on germ cells, then the frequency of dizygotic twinning should be related to maternal age through 'autoaggressive statistics'. Fig. 11.5 supports this contention, although it reveals a complication. The points should rise continuously to a plateau. Instead, they fall off in the highest age group. This suggests that the relative fertility of mothers predisposed to dizygotic twinning declines above the age of about 35 years.

If maternal genes predisposing to dizygotic twinning are associated with pleiotropic effects – and the connection with Klinefelter's syndrome suggests they are – some potential difficulties arise for genetic studies. Dizygotic twins may be more predisposed to some diseases, and less predisposed to others, than monozygotic twins. In certain situations, misleading concordances might well result. As a safeguard, the absolute prevalence or onset-rates of diseases should be assessed both in monozygotic and dizygotic twins as well as in the general population.

In summary, highly complex associations exist between familial autoaggressive diseases of the thyroid and pancreas, chromosomal abnormalities, dizygotic twinning, and acute childhood leukaemia. Nevertheless, the welter of observations

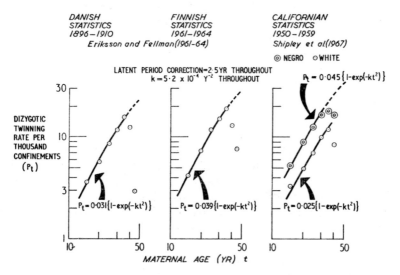

Fig. 11.5 Frequency of dizygotic twinning as a function of maternal age. Danish statistics, 1896 to 1910; and Finnish statistics, 1961–64; from Eriksson and Fellman (1967). Californian statistics from Shipley *et al.* (1967). (The frequency of monozygotic twinning is independent of maternal age.) In all the data, the age-frequency for dizygotic twinning follows autoaggressive statistics over a limited age range only: from $t = 15$ to about 35 years of age. Departures from the theoretical curves above $t = 35$ years suggest that, above this age, women predisposed to dizygotic twinning become relatively less fertile than women in the general population. Another auto-aggressive condition probably competes with autoaggressive-induced dizygotic twinning. Because women with the relevant forbidden-clone will not always produce dizygotic twins, the value of S will be proportional to, but not equal to the size of the sub-group of women at risk with respect to dizygotic twinning. The value of S is lowest (0.025) in the Californian white, and highest (0.045) in the Californian negro population. Note the striking consistency of latent periods and k values for series from three different countries, for whites and Negroes, and at periods ranging from 1896 to 1964.

can be subsumed under one general theory: each of the con-
ditions mentioned has an autoaggressive aetiology, and the positive associations between different conditions can be attributed to predisposing pleiotropic genes. Given adequate

statistics for a defined population, the nature and the frequency of the predisposing genes could be calculated. Anomalies involving the X chromosome are often connected with auto-aggressive disorders. I have concluded from age-pattern and genetic analysis that X-linked genes contribute to the patho-genesis of many autoaggressive diseases. Genetic predisposition, and somatic mutations that initiate these disorders, often implicate X-linked genes. The cytogenetic observations further emphasise the key role of the X chromosome.

BURKITT'S LYMPHOMA AND HODGKIN'S DISEASE. AGE AND
ANATOMICAL DISTRIBUTIONS

The sex- and age-distributions of Burkitt's lymphoma of the jaws (Adatia 1966) and of Hodgkin's disease (Registrar General 1958) are shown in Figs 11.6 and 11.7. They conform satis-factorily to statistics of autoaggressive disease, and they indicate that both diseases are genetically-based. At least two distinctive genotypes appear to be implicated in each disease. (The very few adult-onset cases of Burkitt's lymphoma are not plotted in Fig. 11.6; they may arise in one or more other genotypes, or they may result from an exceptionally long latent period.) Latent periods are the same in males and females both in Hodgkin's disease and in Burkitt's lymphoma, and hence the primary 'autoantibodies' are likely to be humoral (? α_2-globulins).

When we examine the anatomical distribution of Burkitt's lymphoma among the four quadrants of the jaws (Adatia 1966) we find this is extremely non-random. Thus, in 163 patients only one side of the mandible or maxilla was affected; in thirty-nine patients two quadrants were affected; in seven patients three were; but in forty-one patients all four quadrants were involved. This distribution, together with the further details given in Adatia's (1966) paper, suggests by analogy with the arguments in Chapter 8, that the siting of lymphomas of the jaws is determined by multiple MCP–TCF genes.

It is not yet clear whether Hodgkin's disease is unicentric or multicentric in origin, but Rosenberg and Kaplan (1966) favour the view that it arises in a single focus and spreads in a predictable manner along adjacent lymphoid channels. I find their arguments unconvincing, and the opposite conclusions of Smithers (1967) persuasive. Their own evidence, together with that of Smithers (1967), seems to favour the view that the

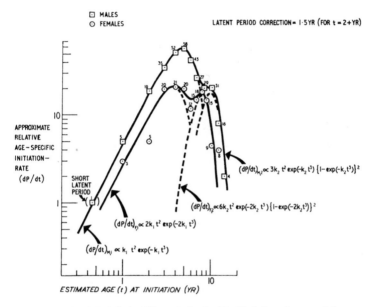

BURKITT'S TUMOUR IN UGANDA. 1953-1965 | *FROM ADATIA (1966)*

Fig. 11.6 Adatia's (1966) statistics for Burkitt's lymphoma of the jaws, in Uganda 1953 to 1965. For initiation in the 0 to 14 years age-range, two genetically-distinctive groups can be discerned. In the early onset-group (initiation modes: 3·8 years females; 4·8 years males), three dependent-type events are needed to initiate the disease ($r = 3$), and one of them is X-linked. The k values for this group are 6×10^{-3} yr^{-3} (males), and $1·2 \times 10^{-2}$ yr^{-3} (females). For the late onset-group (initiation modes: 8·1 years females; 10·2 years males), three independent sets of three dependent-type initiating events appear to be needed ($n = 3$; $r = 3$), and one event in each set is X-linked. For this group, k_M is $1·35 \times 10^{-3}$ yr^{-3}, and k_F is $2·7 \times 10^{-3}$ yr^{-3}. Normalising the size ($S_{1,F}$) of the group of females predisposed to the early onset form of the disease to 1·0, the relative sizes of the other predisposed groups are: $S_{2,F} = 1·1$; $S_{1,M} = 3·4$; and $S_{2,M} = 2·1$. Hence, sex-linked as well as autosomal factors are involved in the polygenic predisposing genotypes.

disease is often multicentric in origin, and that the lymph nodes affected are determined, at least in the early stages, by genetic factors. Not one of the 100 untreated patients examined by Rosenberg and Kaplan (1966) had only one affected lymph node, and bilateral symmetry of neck gland involvement was found in fifty-six of these patients.

Hence, the age- and the anatomical-distributions, both of

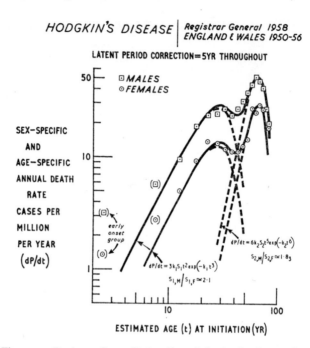

Fig. 11.7 Registrar General's (1958) statistics for death rates from Hodgkin's disease in England and Wales, 1950 to 1956. Similar bimodal age-patterns are found in U.S. and Danish statistics (MacMahon 1966). Suggestions of an early onset-group, with mortality predominantly in the 0 to 9 years age-range, are present in these England and Wales, and also in U.S. statistics (Miller 1966). For the group with a modal initiation-age at 28 years, $r = 3$; $k_1 \simeq 3 \cdot 0 \times 10^5 \, \mathrm{yr}^{-3}$; $S_{1,M} \simeq 7 \cdot 5 \times 10^{-4}$; $S_{1,F} \simeq 3 \cdot 5 \times 10^{-4}$. The late onset group, with modal initiation at about 65 years, is characterised by: $r = 6$; $k_2 \simeq 1 \cdot 1 \times 10^{-11} \, \mathrm{yr}^{-6}$; $S_{2,M} \simeq 1 \cdot 6 \times 10^{-3}$; $S_{2,F} \simeq 8 \cdot 7 \times 10^{-4}$. Genetic predisposition to the early- and late-onset forms of the disease involves both sex-linked and autosomal factors.

Burkitt's lymphoma of the jaws, and of Hodgkin's disease, support the autoaggressive interpretation. The remarkable regressions of Burkitt's lymphoma that have been observed (Burkitt *et al.* 1965) and the ready response, both of this lymphoma and of Hodgkin's disease to chemotherapy and radiotherapy, become more intelligible if they are autoaggressive diseases, rather than 'true' cancers arising from aberrations of TCF synthesis.

But as with the phenomena of the leukaemias, the key question we have to raise is the nature of the target tissue. Lymphocytes and histiocytes which make up the bulk of the tissue in lymph nodes affected by Hodgkin's disease are not malignant, and only the abnormal reticular cells of the Reed-Sternberg type are regarded as neoplastic (Rubin 1966). These reticular cells are likely to be the target of the primary autoaggressive attack.

BIOLOGICAL INTERPRETATION

We have proposed that afferent TCFs are 'processed' by reticular or macrophagic cells in lymph nodes before being presented to mitotic control cells (Ballantyne and Burwell 1965; Burch and Burwell 1965). The biological function of processed TCFs is twofold: firstly they are required to promote mitosis of the lymphoid and myeloid series of growth-control effector cells to provide the necessary amplification in the negative-feedback circuit; and secondly, they are required in the peripheral feedback loop to inhibit the release of humoral or cellular MCPs in the mature form needed to stimulate symmetrical mitosis (Burch and Burwell 1965). Variations in the concentration of TCFs around the normal 'working-point' are therefore followed by variations, of the *opposite phase*, in the release of effector MCPs. (This is *negative* feedback.) Below a critical concentration level, processed TCFs will, however, fail to maintain amplification, and the output of MCPs will then fall off with a further lowering in the concentration of processed TCFs.

We also argued that the overall control of growth probably involves a series of feedback loops, and, in the case of the lymphoid system at least, the first 'relay station' appears to be the thymus, the second being regional lymph nodes (Fig. 11.8). The complete chain of growth-control by lymphoid elements probably involves three species of affector TCFs: from the target tissue, the lymph nodes, and the thymus; as well as three sets of processing cells: in the lymph nodes, thymus, and bone marrow respectively. (See Fig. 11.8.)

Cells processing TCFs in the bone marrow, thymus, and lymph nodes are all 'target-cells' from the viewpoint of growth-control. In the appropriate genotype(s), according to our theory these processing cells will be susceptible to autoaggressive disease. What then would be the consequence of such an attack? Suppose TCF-processing cells in a regional lymph node are attacked. Initially, the supply of processed TCFs to the growth

POSSIBLE STATIONS IN THE HOMOEOSTATIC CONTROL OF GROWTH

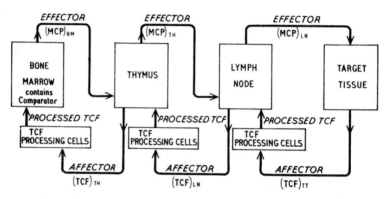

Fig. 11.8 A series of feedback loops connects the comparator in the bone marrow to the target tissue. Whether the thymus participates in growth-control by the granulocytic series is unknown. Tissue mast cells may sometimes provide the ultimate control stage (instead of the lymph node) for humoral MCPs. Autoaggressive damage to TCF processing cells, at any stage, will disturb the release of effector MCPs.

control cells in this node will be reduced, and hence the target-tissue supplying the TCFs will 'appear' to be too small. An enhanced rate of release of mitogenic effectors will follow, to produce (transient) hyperplasia of target tissues. With increasing severity of the autoaggressive attack on the TCF-processing cells, the supply of processed TCFs will be unable to sustain full amplification of the growth-control series in the lymph node. When the effectors are lymphocytes, they will be released in an immature form incapable of stimulating mitosis. If most of the processing cells are rendered ineffectual by the primary autoaggressive attack, the supply of processed TCFs will be so drastically reduced that no lymphoid effectors – mature or immature – will be released. A lymphopenia will result, although the lymph node will be congested with immature lymphocytes.

This analysis predicts therefore: (i) a clinical course characteristic of autoaggressive disease, showing remissions and exacerbations; (ii) spreading of the disease will be associated with a progressive disturbance in delayed hypersensitivity reactions, and a reduced ability to reject skin grafts, because both these phenomena depend upon mature growth-control lymphocytes; and (iii) raised levels of circulating immature lymphocytes during the early stages of the disease followed by reduced levels (lymphopenia) and hypogammaglobulinaemia (see Chapter 9) during the terminal stages. All these predictions are confirmed where Hodgkin's disease is concerned (see, for example, Rubin 1966; Ultmann et al. 1966; Leader Brit. Med. J., 6 May 1967; Smithers 1967). I propose, therefore, that Hodgkin's disease represents an autoaggressive attack on TCF-processing cells in lymph nodes.

A lymphoproliferative disorder could equally well arise if the target cells of the autoaggressive attack were the processing cells serving the immunoglobulin cell series (see Chapter 9). In such an attack, the feedback control over the proliferation of cells synthesising immunoglobulins will be destroyed, with the result that these lymphoid cells will multiply without restraint. Certain cell lines cultured from Burkitt's lymphoma have in fact been found to synthesise immunoglobulins (Fahey et al. 1966; Hinuma and Grace 1967; Minowada et al. 1967; Klein et al. 1967) and hence this tumour might arise from an autoaggressive attack on cells that process immunoglobulins. Myelomatous disease might result from an attack on one or more sets of immunoglobulin-processing cells in the bone marrow.

Suppose reticular cells which process TCFs in the bone marrow become the targets of autoaggressive disease. A reduction in the supply of processed TCFs will remove the restraints from the release of lymphoid or granulocytic growth-control cells. Clones of immature lymphoid or granulocyte-series cells will then be propagated. In other words, a leukaemia will develop from multiple stem cells. When TCF processing cells become severely damaged, the supply of processed TCFs may fail to maintain amplification in the growth-control series, and an aleukaemic leukaemia, with a reduced level of circulating leucocytes will result.

However, there are several indications that chronic myeloid leukaemia may be monoclonal in origin (Fialkow *et al.* 1967). If these indications are confirmed, a different pathogenetic mechanism will have to be invoked for this type of leukaemia. I have maintained that an endogenous defence mechanism normally comes into operation to attempt to suppress the auto-antigenic forbidden-clone, and that defence is mediated through immunoglobulins. In Chapter 9, I argued that the classical immune response involves at least two main groups of cells. Lymphoid and plasma cells synthesise the several types of immunoglobulin antibodies, while processing cells (reticular cells and macrophages) ingest the antigen-antibody complex and then process the antibody for presentation to the antibody-synthesising cells. Both groups of cells are target cells from the viewpoint of growth-control and therefore in the appropriate genotypes, both are potential victims of autoaggressive attacks. When a forbidden-clone arises which attacks either type of defence cell, a vicious situation is created where the efficiency of defence is grossly impaired. Consequently, the forbidden-clone will then proliferate in a relatively unrestricted manner to give rise to a monoclonal leukaemia. However, Morley *et al.* (1967) have observed two patients with chronic myeloid leukaemia in whom leucocyte counts showed a gross and apparently spontaneous oscillation. This periodic behaviour suggests that high rates of proliferation from the mutant stem cell will tend to diminish the output of mature primary ($\alpha_2 M$) autoantibodies. The subsequent recovery of the defence system could then restrain the proliferation of the forbidden-clone and bring about an oscillation in the level of circulating leucocytes.

Our arguments concerning autoaggressive attacks on TCF-processing cells should be relevant to the nature of thymomas. Significantly, only a few thymic tumours are regarded as malignant; furthermore, they often occur in conjunction with acute lymphoblastic leukaemia (Anderson and Pederson 1967). The histopathology of thymic tumours frequently reveals large numbers of epithelial cells (Hale and Scowen 1967). These cells may normally process TCFs from lymph nodes.

Autoaggressive damage to processing cells may be responsible for many proliferative disorders.

DO VIRUSES HAVE AN AETIOLOGICAL ROLE?

The complicity of viruses in the aetiology of leukaemia, Burkitt's lymphoma, and Hodgkin's disease is often alleged, and epidemiological evidence for a viral cause for Burkitt's lymphoma looks persuasive. However, Seldam *et al.* (1966) find it difficult to believe that a specific virus occurs in tropical Africa and New Guinea, where Burkitt's lymphoma is common, and not in intervening countries with similar climatic conditions, where the tumour is unknown. The occurrence of the disease in Denmark, the United Kingdom, and South and North America (Jensen 1967) has also to be explained.

Fig. 11.6 suggests that Burkitt's tumour of the jaws is basically autoaggressive in aetiology, and that it is confined to specific genotypes in which sex-linked as well as autosomal factors are implicated. Gene frequencies may therefore account for some features of the geographical distribution of the disease. The number of cases of childhood lymphoma in Papua and New Guinea reported by Seldam *et al.* (1966) is small, but their sex- and age-distributions bear a striking resemblance to those in Fig. 11.6. Because the relatively abundant data for males in Uganda fit autoaggressive statistics so accurately, the random initiating events are most unlikely to be viral infections. If a virus is involved in this disease it probably affects the progression phase. Infective agents (bacteria as well as viruses), can often act as precipitating and exacerbating factors in autoaggressive disease (see Chapter 9). Agents of this kind can therefore be expected to precipitate the symptomatic and clinical onset of leukaemias, Burkitt's lymphoma, and Hodgkin's disease. We need to determine whether such agents – specific or relatively non-specific – are *essential* to their onset. Is the forbidden-clone eliminated or perpetually suppressed by the host's defence mechanism in the absence of interference by certain micro-organisms – and notably by viruses?

To explore this question, we need among other things to analyse the sex- and age-distributions of diseases in which viruses indubitably play a necessary aetiological role.

AGE-DISTRIBUTIONS OF VIRAL DISEASES

Poliomyelitis

Greenberg's (1965) data for an epidemic of poliomyelitis in New York City, 1949–50, are illustrated in Fig. 11.9. Age-

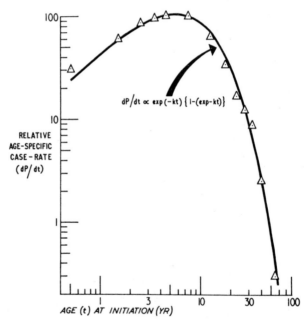

Fig. 11.9   Greenberg's (1965) data for cases of poliomyelitis, New York City 1949 to 1950. The theoretical curve is $dP/dt \propto \exp(-kt)$ $\{1 - \exp(-kt)\}$, with $k \simeq 0.13$ yr^{-1}. It could be interpreted to mean that the development of lesions requires the presence of two independent forbidden-clones in addition to the poliomyelitis virus. The very short latent period suggests that the second clone has to be initiated either shortly before, or during, the viral infection. From the statistics for males and females separately, the ratio of predisposed males to females (S_M/S_F) is about 1.3.

specific case-rates give an excellent fit to autoaggressive statistics. If complications from natural immunity and other causes can be neglected, then two independent and distinctive clones are needed to initiate clinically-detectable signs of polio-myelitis in predisposed and infected individuals. However, if natural immunity was present in some people, this could complicate the interpretation because it might add an age-dependent factor; the actual risk of being infected by the virus might add yet another such factor. If despite these possible complications the simplest interpretation is valid, then the latent period is very short – much less than one year, at least in infants and children.

This suggests that the lesions of poliomyelitis develop only when the second forbidden-clone has been initiated either shortly prior to, or during, an infection with the poliomyelitis virus. In the absence of the virus, the host normally suppresses, or eliminates, the forbidden-clone; in the absence of the forbidden-clone, the virus is eventually eliminated by the host's immune defence apparatus.

This new approach accounts for the contribution of genetic factors to infectious diseases and the well-known *carrier state*. In this state, a person carries an infective agent, such as the poliomyelitis virus, without showing the symptoms and signs of the disease seen in vulnerable people.

Infectious hepatitis

Age-distributions of infectious hepatitis (Fig. 11.10) point to a similar interpretation. Here, three genetically-predisposed groups are at risk, and an average latent period of about six months intervenes between the initiation of the forbidden-clone and the precipitation of the onset of disease by the infecting virus.

Mumps

Some impressive epidemiological data for mumps (Witte and Karchmer 1968) strongly support our proposal that an auto-aggressive component underlies the pathogenesis of various infectious diseases. Relative age-specific onset-rates of cases from selected areas of the United States fit autoaggressive statistics very precisely (see Fig. 11.11). The average latent period between the initiation of the forbidden-clone (or the last forbidden-clone) and the appearance of symptoms is very short: 0·1 per year or less. Disease manifestations evidently

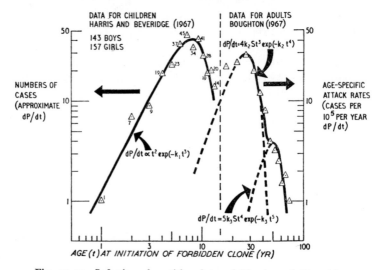

Fig. 11.10 Infectious hepatitis: data of Harris and Beveridge (1967) for children, and of Boughton (1967) for higher age ranges. Three predisposed groups can be discerned. For the early onset group with initiation mode at 7·8 years, the value of r is 3; $k_1 \simeq 1\cdot4 \times 10^{-3}$ yr^{-3}; and $\lambda = 0\cdot5$ year. The second group, with initiation mode at 27 years is characterised by: $r = 4$; $k_2 \simeq 1\cdot4 \times 10^{-6}$ yr^{-4}; $\lambda \sim 0\cdot5$ year. For the late onset group $r = 5$; $k_3 \simeq 2\cdot6 \times 10^{-9}$ yr^{-5}; $\lambda \sim 0\cdot5$ year.

depend on the virus being present in the victim at the time of, or shortly after the occurrence of the last initiating somatic mutation. Moreover, the persistence of the active disease process probably depends on the continued presence of the infecting agent. When the classical immune and phagocytic systems have succeeded in combating the viral infection, they are then freed to suppress the forbidden-clone. In a disease such as poliomyelitis, permanent disability results because neurons cannot be regenerated, and not because nerve tissue continues to be destroyed.

When the latent period is very short, we might expect the disease to be rare. We might argue that the chance of being infected within a month or so of the emergence of a forbidden-clone must be small. On the contrary, we know that a

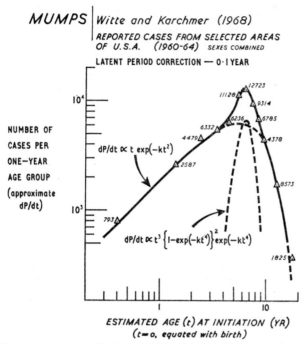

MUMPS | *Witte and Karchmer (1968)*

REPORTED CASES FROM SELECTED AREAS
OF U.S.A. (1960-64) *SEXES COMBINED*

LATENT PERIOD CORRECTION — 0·1 YEAR

NUMBER OF CASES PER ONE—YEAR AGE GROUP (approximate dP/dt)

$dP/dt \propto t \exp(-kt^2)$

$dP/dt \propto t^3 \left\{1-\exp(-kt^4)\right\}^2 \exp(-kt^4)$

ESTIMATED AGE (t) AT INITIATION (YR)
(t=0, equated with birth)

Fig. 11.11 Age-specific data, combined for sex, for reported cases of mumps from selected areas of the United States (Los Angeles County, excluding Los Angeles City; New York City; and Milwaukee and Madison, Wisconsin) for the period 1960 to 1964 (Witte and Karchmer 1968). Two predisposed groups with onset before 20 years of age can be detected. Details of the 6 per cent of all cases with adult onset (20 years and over) were not given, but at least one further predisposed group exists. The slight misfit of the point at $t = 17.4$ years might indicate a contribution from such a group. A latent period correction of 0·1 year has been applied throughout, on the assumption that zero age can be equated with birth. Alternatively, the latent period could be still shorter, if 'zero age' ($t = 0$) commences up to 0·1 year prior to birth. Relative age-specific initiation-rates, dP/dt, for the majority of early-onset cases fit the equation: $dP/dt \propto t \exp(-k_1 t^2)$, with $k_1 = 1.7 \times 10^{-2}$ yr^{-2}. The curve for the small group giving a mode at $t = 6.4$ year, is probably defined by: $dP/dt \propto t^3 \exp(-k_2 t^4)$. $\{1-\exp(-k_2 t)^4\}^2$. If this is correct, then three forbidden-clones are required to produce mumps in this genotype; the growth of each clone is initiated by four somatic mutations in a single growth-control stem cell.

substantial proportion of the population has had an attack of mumps.

To reconcile these apparent contradictions, and to explain the excellent conformity of the age-distribution of mumps

(Fig. 11.11) to autoaggressive statistics, we have to postulate the existence in genetically-predisposed persons of multiple sets of similar, but not identical, growth-control stem cells. Each set can yield a forbidden-clone which, in the presence of the infecting virus, will give rise to an attack of mumps. (This situation resembles that discussed in connection with dental caries in Chapter 8. The growth of each of the many distinctive sets of odontoblasts is regulated by its own central growth-control element. Excepting molars, the kinetics of forbidden-clone initiation are similar for attacks of dental caries on all types of permanent teeth.) In the main group of people pre-disposed to mumps, the kinetics of the initiation of a forbidden-clone from each distinctive set of growth-control stem cells, is described by: $dP/dt = 2kt \exp(-kt^2)$, where k is 1.7×10^{-2} yr^{-2} for each set of stem cells at mutant risk.

I should add that this new approach to the pathogenesis of infectious diseases readily accounts for their anatomical specificity. It also illustrates the complexity of pathology. Considerable discretion should be exercised when speaking of the 'cause' of a disease.

Statistics of epidemics

Autoaggressive diseases with a very short latent period and an essential contribution from an infective agent show character-istic epidemic statistics. Marked fluctuations of incidence are seen from season to season, and from year to year. In Witte and Karchmer's (1968) study of mumps, a low of fifty cases per 100 000 population was recorded in 1922 and a high of 250 cases per 100 000 was found in 1941. The graph of yearly incidence-rate against year follows an extremely erratic, zig-zag course. In 1965, some forty-two cases were reported from selected areas in May, and only ten in September (Witte and Karchmer 1968). The monthly case-rate fluctuates as erratic-ally as the yearly case-rate.

In contrast, when we study a classical 'autoimmune' disease such as chronic discoid lupus erythematosus, we find a striking constancy in the yearly incidence-rate. From November 1958 to November 1966 the numbers of new cases seen each year in the Department of Dermatology, at the Leeds General Infirmary, has varied between the surprisingly narrow limits of twenty-seven and thirty-four (Burch and Rowell 1968).

Burkitt's lymphoma, leukaemia, Hodgkin's disease and infective agents

If these proliferative diseases are triggered by an infective agent, and if such an agent is necessary to their development, then clear-cut evidence for epidemics should be obtainable. Lee (1962) has found a statistically-significant seasonal variation in the onset of lymphocytic-, but not myeloid-leukaemia, for the age-range 0 to 19 years. However, early suggestions that leukaemia cases sometimes cluster in time and space have not withstood rigorous statistical analysis (Ederer *et al.* 1964), although a slight tendency to space-time clustering has been reported recently (Till *et al.* 1967). When a disease is genetically-based, space-time clustering needs to be assessed in relation to the distribution of predisposing genes. Consequently, the evidence for the space-time clustering of Burkitt's tumour (Pike *et al.* 1967) is difficult to interpret, but the finding of possible low- and high-risk areas may reflect in part an uneven distribution of genetically-predisposed individuals.

The inability so far (1967) to recover consistently a specific infective agent from patients with these diseases constitutes only weak evidence against the view that micro-organisms are essential aetiological factors. Such an agent may always be found in the future. MacMahon and Levy (1964) find a concordance-rate for childhood leukaemia of probably more than 25 per cent in monozygotic twins, but probably less than 100 per cent. At first sight this seems to favour an essential environmental contribution to the multifactorial pathogenesis of leukaemia. However, Fig. 11.2 reveals a major complication with respect to penetrance in relation to leukaemia type. Whereas the penetrance of the two early-onset forms of acute lymphatic leukaemia is nearly 100 per cent by 12 years of age, the average penetrance of acute myeloid and monocytic leukaemias appears to be much less than 100 per cent during childhood. Suppose after careful follow-up, and correction for inter-current mortality, concordance-rates in monozygotic twins for the early onset forms of acute lymphatic leukaemia during childhood were found to be less than 100 per cent.

Then, very serious consideration would have to be given to an essential aetiological role for environmental factors.

Other evidence which might implicate infective agents concerns birth-order. Several investigators have shown that in large families, the first-born have a higher risk of leukaemia than their later-born sibs (Stewart *et al.* 1958; Manning and Carroll 1957; MacMahon and Newill 1962; Stark and Mantel 1966). This birth-order effect might be explained if the later-born are immunised very early in life through the infections brought into the family by their older sibs. When the forbidden-clone appears in the later-born, these sibs will often be pre-immunised against the triggering leukaemogenic micro-organisms. On this view, the leukaemic risk should decline progressively with increasing order in the sibship. Unfortunately the precise assessment of risk is complicated by an independent effect – that of maternal age. For a given place in the sibship order, the leukaemic risk increases with maternal age. Correcting for the maternal age effect, Stark and Mantel (1966) find that the risk of leukaemia is approximately constant for the first three children in a sibship, but it falls off for the fourth- and fifth-born. Moreover, they find the birth-order effect (and also the maternal-age effect) is most important for leukaemias producing death in the 10 to 15 years age group. Hence, these two influences on leukaemic risk may be largely or wholly confined to monocytic and myeloid leukaemias. If Stark and Mantel's (1966) findings are confirmed, then the quantitative features of the birth-order effect might be explained if those mothers giving birth to children developing monocytic or myeloid leukaemias are, on the average, less fertile than other mothers in the general population. This hypothesis could be tested by epidemiological studies.

Summarising, none of the available evidence for childhood leukaemia, Burkitt's lymphoma, or Hodgkin's disease compels us to assume that micro-organisms play anything other than a precipitating role in the pathogenesis of these diseases. They may shorten the latent period, and thus give some indications of space-time clustering, but in their absence, these diseases may still manifest themselves, although later. However, definite conclusions cannot be drawn from this ill-defined situation. Readers in search of a more optimistic account may wish to consult the writings of Bryan *et al.* (1967) and Rous (1967).

On surer ground, the sex-, age-, and (where relevant) anatomical distributions leave little doubt that genetic factors, somatic mutations, and forbidden-clones make essential intrinsic contributions to the pathogenesis of these proliferative diseases. From the biological viewpoint, Hodgkin's disease, lymphosarcomas, reticulosarcomas, thymomas, and the several types of leukaemia may well furnish valuable insights into the mechanism of normal growth-control.

12. REFLECTIONS

*'It is clear that a comprehensive view, synoptic in character, is necessary –
as Plato maintained – if whatever total knowledge is accessible to us is
not to be partly lost through specialist fragmentation.'*

F. I. G. Rawlins, 1965

In this book, two major biological concepts have been tested
and elaborated by analysing age-patterns and anatomical
distributions of disease. Concept (1), introduced by Burwell
in 1963, is fundamental to the physiology of multi-tissue
organisms; and concept (2), proposed by Burnet in 1959, is
fundamental to much of their pathology.

(1) From the study of cellular reactions in lymph nodes to
tissue transplants, and from general biological considerations,
Burwell proposed that the growth of mammals is centrally
regulated by the lymphoid system. One class of small lymphocytes from this system probably stimulates symmetrical mitosis
in certain target cells. Many tissues, however, lie behind blood-
tissue barriers, and a parallel system, utilising humoral mitogenic effectors controls the growth of such tissues. In mammals,
the humoral growth-control effectors may prove to be α_2-
macroglobulins. Basophilic granulocytes and mast cells appear
to be responsible for their production.

(2) From broad immunological considerations, Burnet
reasoned that 'autoimmune' diseases could result from a *central*
breakdown in self-tolerance. Gene change in a mesenchymal
stem cell could initiate the growth of a clone – the 'forbidden-
clone' – of mutant cells synthesising cellular or humoral autoantibodies. These autoantibodies circulate in the body fluids
to attack and damage target cells bearing complementary
antigens: symptoms and signs of disease follow.

I conclude that the mesenchymal stem cells, capable when
mutant of propagating forbidden-clones, act normally as
central comparators in the feedback control of growth. When

the results of experiment and observation are coupled with theory, it appears that immunoglobulin autoantibodies cannot be the *primary* pathogenic agents in 'autoimmune' disease. Accordingly, the term 'autoimmune' disease, which for many people connotes disturbances in immunoglobulin antibody production that are causally related to the disease, has been replaced here by the less misleading, and more apt expression: *autoaggressive* disease.

Additions and modifications of detail excepted, I have maintained that the seminal ideas of Burnet and Burwell are essentially correct, and that through their amalgamation and extension, a far-ranging biological synthesis can be formulated. Unfortunately, the would-be synthesiser is obliged to survey fields in which he has no specialist training, and he cannot always distinguish, even with the help of specialists, that which is scientifically established from that which is mythology and dogma. Of course there are compensating advantages inasmuch as the non-specialist often brings a new outlook, and new techniques, to bear an old problems.

CONTROL AND CO-ORDINATION OF GROWTH

Looking back on the crucial problem of explaining co-ordinated growth in metazoa, it seems to me that in a rational approach, we first have to decide whether the growth of a specific tissue is regulated by a mechanism intrinsic to that tissue, or whether a homoeostatic device is used, with an external or 'central' control. Experimental evidence reviewed in Chapter 6 shows that in mice and/or rats, normal growth, regenerative growth of the liver, and compensatory growth of the kidney are 'centrally' controlled. Factors essential to growth are provided by lymphoid tissue and bone marrow. However, the important distinction (Chapter 2) between symmetrical and asymmetrical mitosis has to be remembered; the form of growth with which we are concerned here involves symmetrical mitosis.

Once the principle of the central control of growth is accepted, the next problem to tackle is that of recognition. How does the effector signal – the *mitotic control protein* or MCP from the central organ – identify the target tissue (characterised by a *tissue coding factor* or TCF); and how does the affector from the target tissue – related to the TCF – find its central control organ?

When we reflect upon our own incredible biological complexity (look again at your finger-prints), and when we realise that different organs follow different growth curves, the recognition problem assumes terrifying proportions – especially when we remember that it arises at both the central and the peripheral ends of the feedback control loop. In Chapter 6, I argued that only one genetic and molecular basis for mutual MCP–TCF recognition, at both ends of the feedback loop is feasible. The genes that code in a given individual for some or all of the protein components of a specific central recognition molecule (MCP), are the same as those which code in target cells for the comparable protein components of the cognate peripheral recognition molecule (TCF). In other words, some or all of the polypeptide chains of a given MCP, in a given individual, are identical with the corresponding polypeptide chains of the cognate TCF. The distinction between humoral MCPs and humoral TCFs resides in their non-protein components. Although I first derived these conclusions from a theoretical analysis of some unexpectedly simple features in the age-distributions of autoaggressive disease, I subsequently fortified them by a more direct argument based on independent biological considerations.

Homoeostatic control requires a stable comparator in the central system whereby the size of the target tissue can be measured. Analysis of the age-distributions of autoaggressive diseases indicates that this comparator is supplied by a fixed number of growth-control stem cells. The growth of each distinctive target tissue is regulated by its own comparator. Co-ordination of growth is based on the fixed relations between the number of stem cells in any one growth-control element, and all other such elements.

THE PATHOGENESIS OF DEGENERATIVE DISEASE

If the primary question in co-ordinated growth-control concerns the location of the controlling system, what then is the paramount issue raised by degenerative disease and ageing? It relates, of course, to the nature of the pathogenic mechanism:

Is it a stochastic (random) process? Or, like development and growth, is it deterministic and sequential? Or is it partly stochastic and partly deterministic? A vast repository of scarcely-tapped data for age-distributions shows, beyond reasonable doubt, that autoaggressive diseases, which include many ageing conditions, are initiated by random events. These events occur in growth-control stem cells, the number of which is constant from around, or before birth, to the end of the life-span. The stem cells comprise the growth-control comparator. (There is a nice antithesis between the rigorously defined number of growth-control stem cells – the outcome of an orderly developmental process – and the randomness of the chaos-producing errors which subsequently occur in these cells.)

Aetiological studies are plagued by intricate problems of cause and effect. Changes associated with disease processes are often so numerous that it becomes exceedingly difficult to disentangle the causal chain: indeed, the chain may even transmute into a spiral. In taking his clinical notes, the doctor will give special attention to those unusual events that im-mediately precede the onset of disease, but the question: Have you had any pertinent somatic mutations recently? cannot be readily answered, even when the patient is an expert immunologist. The clinician may find inflammation, the bio-chemist may detect abnormal enzyme or cholesterol levels, the cytogeneticist may see chromosomal abnormalities, and the immunologist may uncover autoantibodies in the IgM or IgG fractions, but as we have heard before, association does not necessarily imply cause. Recently, the tools for investigating disease have ramified . . . 'with the result that time, energy, and money are too often squandered on the trivial, the irrele-vant, and the obvious. The need for thought, observation, ideas, and hypotheses – the hard work of science – recedes'. (Leader, *Brit. Med. J.*, 25 November 1967.)

Among the labyrinthine pathways of pathology, the sex- and age-distributions, and the anatomical siting of lesions provide us with immensely valuable guides if only we can spare time to ponder their significance. When we find, as we frequently do, that the age-distributions of disease after disease conform to Yule statistics, or Weibull statistics, or a combina-tion of the two (see Chapter 4) we can conclude with some confidence that such diseases are initiated by random events. When we discover that a particular random event occurs at an average rate that is unvarying from birth to death, from country to country, and from continent to continent; when we find that certain events in XX females occur at twice the rate of the corresponding events in XY males; and when we encounter rates in trisomy 21 that are higher than those in normal karyotypes – in the way that is detailed in Chapter 11 – we can conclude, again with some confidence, that the initiating events are a form of gene mutation in somatic cells. Chromosomes X and 21 (or 22?) are evidently among those carrying genes that undergo somatic mutation to initiate autoaggressive disease.

In Chapter 7, I suggested these random initiating events involve a spontaneous switch in messenger RNA transcription from the 'correct' template strand of DNA, over to the complementary, anti-parallel strand. We call this a *DNA strand-switching mutation*: the non-simultaneous utilisation of information from both strands of the double-helix is called *genetic dichotomy*. Although this interpretation agrees with evidence from multiple sources, and leads to simple explanations of intergenic recombination, and many examples of genetic polymorphism and heterozygous fitness, the concept is not yet validated. Nevertheless, it makes some precise predictions, and their testing will either substantiate the strand-switching theory or reveal the correct alternative.

Diseases such as osteoporosis and dental caries show anatomical site-distributions that have not been explained by orthodox aetiological theories. So far as my collaborators and I can see, these distributions cannot be convincingly explained in traditional terms. Our theory stresses the uniqueness both of the TCF of an individual element of tissue, and of the specificity of the 'mutant' MCP (the primary 'autoantibody') for its target TCF. Autoaggressive disease is the consequence of a *unique relationship* between complex macromolecules. Because the primary structure of MCPs and TCFs, both normal and mutant, is coded by genes, it follows that the anatomical distribution of the lesions of autoaggressive disease – as well as general susceptibility – will also be genetically determined. The remarkable regularities in the distribution of affected sites in dental caries, together with twins studies, verify these predictions (Chapter 8).

Genetic dichotomy; the physiological role attributed to MCPs in growth-control; and the pathological role attributed to 'mutant' MCPs in autoaggressive disease, give a straightforward biological explanation of the homograft response. In an outbred population, certain MCPs of the host will almost inevitably be complementary and destructive towards certain TCFs of a transplanted allogeneic tissue or organ. Agreement between theory, and the detailed evidence for the role of cellular and humoral MCPs in growth and disease is extensive. Connections between growth and disease; positive and negative associations between morphology and disease; and corresponding associations between one disease and another, are predicted and observed.

ENVIRONMENTAL FACTORS IN DISEASE AND AGEING

Mathematical analysis of the age-distributions of autoaggressive diseases shows that ordinary environments have little or no effect on the rate of the somatic mutations (DNA strand-switching events) that initiate the disease process. Artificially-high intensities of ionising radiation can probably induce this form of gene change, but there are no indications – so far – that agents other than unphysiologically low temperatures can slow the rate of mutation.

The incidence and prevalence of many autoaggressive diseases frequently vary from country to country, and from district to district within a given country. However, the *shape* of the age-distribution curve for a given disease often remains sensibly constant. In these circumstances, the different levels of disease in the separate populations can often be attributed to differences in the proportions of predisposed individuals. These proportions are determined by the frequencies of predisposing genes, and these in turn are subject to differential selection pressures in dissimilar environments.

When the last initiating somatic mutation has occurred an interval – the latent period – has to elapse before the autoaggressive attack of the proliferating forbidden-clone on the target tissue(s) can generate detectable symptoms or signs.

This is the phase of the disease process where environmental factors can sometimes exert a profound impact. Infectious diseases such as poliomyelitis, and allergic diseases such as hay fever, will only manifest themselves when the appropriate virus or pollen has been acquired from the environment. (These environmental agents will only produce pathogenic complications in susceptible individuals, possessing the appropriate forbidden-clone(s).) More commonly, adverse environments exercise a quantitative, rather than qualitative influence, on autoaggressive disease by shortening the average duration of the latent period. Occasionally, specific environmental factors, such as optimum levels of fluoride in the drinking water, can prolong the latent period in diseases such as dental caries and osteoporosis.

Severe mental stress appears to exacerbate most auto-aggressive diseases and sometimes to precipitate their onset.

Our unified theory defines the relative roles of extrinsic and intrinsic pathogenic factors more precisely than previous aetiological theories. And by emphasising the overwhelming importance of somatic mutation it attracts its share of odium. The natural desire of many investigators to substitute environmental factors for somatic mutations is very understandable, but it does not necessarily conduce to an objective appraisal of the evidence.

SCIENTIFIC THEORIES: DESIDERATA

We ask of a scientific theory first, that it should provide the simplest possible interpretation of established observations, and secondly, that it should make critical predictions. Among many predictions, those in Chapters 6 and 7 concerning the amino acid sequence of polypeptides in related MCPs, TCFs, and 'mutant' MCPs are unusually exact. If biochemical studies verify the predicted relations, the stochastic, genetic, molecular, and cellular foundations of our unified theory will be established with a high degree of certainty. Thirdly, we require a scientific theory to provide insight and understanding. Obviously, it is impossible for me or my collaborators to assess this aspect of our work with detachment, and the reader is left to form his own judgment. We are simply unaware of any other current theory that can account for the quantitative features of the sex- and age-distributions of disease, and for the anatomical distributions of lesions in disorders such as dental caries. With respect to comprehensiveness, even the least generous critic would concede, I hope, that our synopsis is without rival.

We cannot avoid asking of a theory of disease and ageing: What are the prospects for cure and prevention? Various suggestions follow from our synopsis and one therapeutic success has already been scored (see Chapter 9). Nevertheless, if we are correct, the lure – or the threat – of eternal corporeal life can be relegated to the remote future. In any case, the benefits mankind can reasonably expect from present and future medical research are likely to be limited mainly by our incapacity either to feed the world's every growing population or to limit its growth.

Throughout this book I have made fairly liberal use of quotation and it is therefore appropriate that I should end by citing Lord Platt's (1967) reference to some words of William Harvey, for, with Lord Platt 'I know that I have spoken some heresies'. In his Harveian Oration: 'Medical Science: Master or Servant?' delivered at the Royal College of Physicians of London on 18 October 1967, Lord Platt rendered Harvey's Latin thus: 'I fear lest I have mankind at large for my enemies, so much doth wont and custom become a second nature. Doctrine once sown strikes deep its root, and respect for antiquity influences all men. Still the die is cast and my trust is in the love of truth and the candour of cultivated minds.'

REFERENCES

Abercrombie, M. and Ambrose, E. J. 1962. The surface properties of cancer cells: a review. *Cancer Res.* **22**, 525–548.

Adatia, A. K. 1966. Burkitt's tumour in the jaws. *Brit. Dent. J.* **120**, 315–326.

Åkesson, H. O. and Forssman, H. 1966. A study of maternal age in Down's syndrome. *Ann. Hum. Genet. Lond.* **29**, 271–276.

Alffram, P.-A. 1964. An epidemiological study of cervical and trochanteric fractures of the femur in an urban population. *Acta Orthopaedica Scand.* Suppl. 65.

Allansmith, M., McClelland, B. and Butterworth, M. 1967. Stability of human immunoglobulin levels. *Proc. Soc. Exp. Biol. Med.* **125**, 404–407.

Alter, M. 1966. Dermatoglyphic analysis as a diagnostic tool. *Medicine*, **46**, 35–56.

Amkraut, A. A., Garvey, J. S. and Campbell, D. H. 1966. Competition of haptens. *J. Exp. Med.* **124**, 293–306.

Amos, D. B., Hattler, B. G., Hutchin, P., McCloskey, R. and Zmijewski, C. M. 1966. Skin donor selection by leucocyte typing. *Lancet*, **i**, 300–302.

Anderson, V. and Pedersen, H. 1967. Thymoma and acute leukaemia. *Acta Med. Scand.* **182**, 581–590.

Archer, O. K., Sutherland, E. R. and Good, R. A. 1963. Appendix of the rabbit: a homologue of the bursa in the chicken. *Nature, Lond.* **200**, 337–339.

Arnason, U. G., Jankovic, B. D. and Waksman, B. H. 1962. A survey of the thymus and its relation to lymphocytes and immune reactions. *Blood*, **20**, 617–628.

Arquilla, E. R. and Finn, J. 1963. Genetic differences in antibody production to determinant groups on insulin. *Science*, **142**, 400–401.

Asboe-Hanson, G. 1964. Dermatologic aspects of mast cell activity. *Dermatologica*, **128**, 51–67.

Ashley, D. J. B. 1967. Observations on the epidemiology of appendicitis. *Gut*, **8**, 533–538.

Atkinson, P. J. and Weatherell, J. A. 1967. Variation in the density of the femoral diaphysis with age. *J. Bone Jt. Surg.* **49B**, 781–788.

Atwell, J. D., Duthie, H. L. and Goligher, J. C. 1965. The outcome of Crohn's disease. *Brit. J. Surg.* **52**, 966–972.

Bailey, D. W. 1963. Histoincompatibility associated with the X chromosome in mice. *Transplantation*, **1**, 70–74.

Ballantyne, B. and Burwell, R. G. 1965. Distribution of cholinesterase in lymph nodes and its possible relation to the regulation of tissue size. *Nature, Lond.* **206**, 1123–1125.

Beckwith, J. R. and Signer, E. R. 1966. Transposition of the *Lac* region of *Escherichia coli*. *J. Mol. Biol.* **19**, 254–265.

Benacerraf, B. 1967. Studies of antigenicity with artificial antigens. In: *Regulation of the Antibody Response*. B. Cinader (ed.). Charles C. Thomas, Springfield, Ill.

Ben-Efraim, S., Fuchs, S. and Sela, M. 1967. Differences in immune response to synthetic antigens in two inbred strains of guinea-pigs. *Immunology*, **12**, 573–581.

Bielický, T., Jezková, Z. and Malina, L. 1966. Tissue antibodies in chronic lupus erythematosus. *Brit. J. Derm.* **78**, 29–33.

Billingham, R. E., Silvers, W. K. and Wilson, D. B. 1965. A second study on the H–Y transplantation antigen in mice. *Proc. Roy. Soc. (Lond.)*, **B163**, 61–89.

Billson, F. A., Dombal, F. T. de, Watkinson, G. and Goligher, J. C. 1967. Ocular complications of ulcerative colitis. *Gut*, **8**, 102–106.

192

Blecher, T. E., Soothill, J. F., Voyce, M. A., and Walker, W. H. C. 1968. Antibody deficiency syndrome: a case with normal immunoglobulin levels. *Clin. exp. Immunol.* **3**, 47–56.

Booth, J. B. and Berry, C. L. 1967. Unilateral pulmonary agenesis. *Arch. Dis. Childh.* **42**, 361–374.

Boughton, C. R. 1967. Viral hepatitis in Sydney: a study of a hospital series. *Med. J. Austr.* **2**, 535–542.

Boyd, E. 1932. The weight of the thymus gland in health and in disease. *Amer. J. Dis. Child.* **43**, 1162–1214.

Boyden, S. V. 1966. Natural antibodies and the immune response. *Adv. Immunol.* **5**, 1–28.

Brand, K. G. 1965. Evolution of specific spectra of immunological responsiveness. *Nature, Lond.* **206**, 1164–1165.

Brenner, S., Stretton, A. O. W. and Kaplan, S. 1965. Genetic code: the 'nonsense' triplets for chain termination and their suppression. *Nature, Lond.* **206**, 994–998.

—— and Milstein, C. 1966. Origin of antibody variability. *Nature, Lond.* **211**, 242–243.

Brewer, G. J., Gall, J. C., Honeyman, M., Gershowitz, H., Shreffler, D. C., Dern, R. J. and Hames, C. 1967. Inheritance of quantitative expression of erythrocyte glucose-6-phosphate dehydrogenase activity in the Negro – a twin study. *Biochem. Genet.* **1**, 41–53.

Brienl, F. and Haurowitz, F. 1930. Chemische unterushung des präzipitates aus hamaglobin unt anti-hämaglobin-serum und bemerkungen über die natur der antikörper. *Z. Phys. Chem.* **192**, 45–57.

Brink, R. A. 1960. Paramutation and chromosome organisation. *Q. Rev. Biol.* **35**, 120–137.

Brostoff, S. W. and Ingram, V. M. 1967. Chemical modification of yeast alanine-tRNA with a radioactive carbodiimide. *Science*, **158**, 666–669.

Brues, A. M., Drury, D. R. and Brues, M. C. 1936. A quantitative study of cell growth in regenerating liver. *Arch. Path.* **22**, 658–673.

Bryan, W. R., Dalton, A. J. and Rauscher, F. J. 1967. The viral approach to human leukaemia and lymphoma: its current status. *Progress in Hematology*, **5**, 137–179.

Bucher, N. L. R. 1967. Experimental aspects of hepatic regeneration. *New Engl. J. Med.* **277**, 686–696.

Bullough, W. S. 1965. Mitotic and functional homeostasis: a speculative review. *Cancer Res.* **25**, 1683–1727.

Burch, P. R. J. 1963a. Human cancer: Mendelian inheritance or vertical transmission? *Nature, Lond.* **197**, 1042–1045.

—— 1963b. Carcinogenesis and cancer prevention. *Nature, Lond.* **197**, 1145–1151.

—— 1963c. Autoimmunity: some aetiological aspects. Inflammatory polyarthritis and rheumatoid arthritis. *Lancet*, **1**, 1253–1257.

—— 1964a. Manic depressive psychosis: some new aetiological considerations. *Brit. J. Psychiat.* **110**, 808–817.

—— 1964b. Schizophrenia: some new aetiological considerations. *Brit. J. Psychiat.* **110**, 818–824.

—— 1964c. Involutional psychosis: some new aetiological considerations. *Brit. J. Psychiat.* **110**, 825–829.

—— 1965. Natural and radiation carcinogenesis in man. I. Theory of initiation phase. II. Natural leukaemogenesis: initiation. III. Radiation carcinogenesis. *Proc. Roy. Soc. (Lond.)*, **162B**, 223–287.

—— 1966a. Dupuytren's contracture: an auto-immune disease? *J. Bone Jt. Surg.* **48B**, 312–319.

—— 1966b. Spontaneous auto-immunity. Equations for sex-specific prevalence and initiation-rates. *J. Theoret. Biol.* **12**, 397–409.

—— 1966c. Age- and sex-distributions for some idiopathic non-malignant conditions in man. Some possible implications for growth-control and natural and radiation-induced ageing. In: *Radiation and Ageing*, 117–155. P. J. Lindop and G. A. Sacher (eds.). Taylor and Francis Ltd., London.

Burch, P. R. J. 1967a. Nature's time-scale: degenerative disease in man. *Nature, Lond.* **216,** 298–299.

—— 1967b. Radiation Biophysics. Chapter 11 In: *Principles of Radiation Protection,* 366–397. K. Z. Morgan and J. E. Turner (eds.). John Wiley & Sons, Inc., New York, London, Sydney.

—— 1968a. Huntington's chorea. Age at onset in relation to aetiology and pathogenesis. In: *Handbook of Clinical Neurology,* **6.** P. J. Vinken and G. W. Bruyn (eds.). North-Holland Publishing Co., Amsterdam. In press.

—— 1968b. Genetic aspects of rheumatic and arthritic diseases. In: *University of Edinburgh Pfizer Medical Monographs* 3. *Rheumatic Diseases,* 29–50. J. J. R. Duthie and W. R. M. Alexander (eds.). Edinburgh University Press, Edinburgh.

—— 1968c. Ionizing radiation and life-shortening. In preparation.

—— and Burwell, R. G. 1965. Self and not-self: a clonal induction approach to immunology. *Q. Rev. Biol.* **40,** 252–279.

—— —— 1967. Delayed hypersensitivity. *Lancet,* **1,** 1109–1110.

—— and Jackson, D. 1966a. Periodontal disease and dental caries. *Brit. Dent. J.* **120,** 127–134.

—— —— 1966b. The greying of hair and the loss of permanent teeth considered in relation to an autoimmune theory of ageing. *J. Gerontol.* **21,** 522–528.

—— and Gunz, F. W. 1967. The distribution of the menopausal age in New Zealand. An exploratory study. *N.Z. Med. J.* **66,** 6–10.

—— and Rowell, N. R. 1963. Menarche and menopause. *Lancet,* **2,** 784–785.

—— —— 1965a. Systemic lupus erythematosus: etiological aspects. *Amer. J. Med.* **38,** 793–801.

—— —— 1965b. Psoriasis: aetiological aspects. *Acta derm.-vener. Stockh.* **45,** 366–380.

—— —— 1968. The sex and age distributions of chronic discoid lupus erythematosus in four countries. Possible aetiological and pathogenetic significance. *Acta derm.-vener. Stockh.* **48,** 33–46.

—— —— and Burwell, R. G. 1964. Autoimmunity and chromosomal aberrations. *Lancet,* **2,** 720.

Burkitt, D., Hutt, M. S. R. and Wright, D. H. 1965. The African lymphoma. Preliminary observations on response to therapy. *Cancer,* **18,** 399–410.

Burnet, F. M. 1957. A modification of Jerne's theory of antibody production using the concept of clonal selection. *Austr. J. Sci.* **20,** 67–69.

—— 1959. *The Clonal Selection Theory of Acquired Immunity.* Cambridge University Press, London.

—— 1961. The new approach to immunology. *New Engl. J. Med.* **264,** 24–34.

—— 1963. *The Integrity of the Body.* Oxford University Press, London.

—— 1965. Somatic mutation and chronic disease. *Brit. Med. J.* **1,** 338–342.

Burwell, R. G. 1962. Studies of the primary and secondary immune responses of lymph nodes draining homografts of fresh cancellous bone with particular reference to mechanisms of lymph node reactivity. *Ann. N.Y. Acad. Sci.* **99,** 821–860.

—— 1963. The role of lymphoid tissue in morphostasis. *Lancet,* **2,** 69–74.

—— 1964. Studies in the transplantation of bone. VII. The fresh composite homograft-autograft of cancellous bone. An analysis of factors leading to osteogenesis in marrow transplants and in marrow-containing bone grafts. *J. Bone Jt. Surg.* **46B,** 110–140.

Butterworth, M., McClelland, B. and Allansmith, M. 1967. Influence of sex on immunoglobulin levels. *Nature, Lond.* **214,** 1224–1225.

Calne, R. Y. 1965. Supply and preservation of kidneys. *Brit. Med. Bull.* **21,** 166–170.

Cannon, P. R. 1949. Dietary protein and antimicrobic defense. *Nutr. Rev.* **7,** 161–164.

Caplan, R. M. 1966. Private communication.

Caron, G. A. 1967. The effect of antigens in combination on lymphocyte transformation *in vitro. Int. Arch. Allergy,* **31,** 521–528.

Carrel, A. 1922. Growth-promoting function of leucocytes. *J. Exp. Med.* **36**, 385–391.

Carroll, H. W. and Kimeldorf, D. J. 1967. Protection through parabiosis against the lethal effects of exposure to large doses of X-rays. *Science,* **156**, 954–955.

Centeno, E., Shulman, S., Milgrom, F. and Witebsky, E. 1964. Immunological studies on adrenal glands. VI. The multiple nature of the rabbit adrenal autoantigens. *Immunology,* **8**, 160–169.

Chandler, J. H., Reed, T. E. and De Jong, R. N. 1960. Huntington's chorea in Michigan. *Neurology, Minn.* **10**, 148–153.

Chiba, C., Kondo, M., Rosenblatt, M. and Bing, R. J. 1966. Serum electrophoretic changes following heart allotransplantation. *Proc. Soc. Exp. Biol. Med.* **123**, 746–751.

Clarkson, B., Thompson, D., Horwith, M., and Luckey, E. H. 1960. Cyclical edema and shock due to increased capillary permeability. *Am. J. Med.* **29**, 193–216.

Clawson, C. C., Cooper, M. D. and Good, R. A. 1967. Lymphocyte fine structure in the bursa of Fabricius, the thymus, and the germinal centers. *Laboratory Investigation,* **16**, 407–421.

Cobb, S. and Hall, W. 1965. Newly identified cluster of diseases. *J.A.M.A.* **193**, 1077–1079.

Cohen, S. N. and Hurwitz, J. 1967. Transcription of complementary strands of phage λ DNA *in vivo* and *in vitro. Proc. Nat Acad. Sci. U.S.* **57**, 1759–1766.

Coman, D. R. 1961. Adhesiveness and stickiness: two independent properties of the cell surface. *Cancer Res.* **21**, 1436–1438.

Comfort, A. 1963. Mutation, autoimmunity and ageing. *Lancet,* **2**, 138–141.

—— 1964. *Ageing, the Biology of Senescence.* Second Edition. Routledge and Kegan Paul, London.

Comings, D. E. 1967. The duration of replication of the inactive X chromosome in humans based on the persistence of the heterochromatic sex chromatin body during DNA synthesis. *Cytogenetics,* **6**, 20–37.

Conard, R. A. 1964. Indirect effect of X-radiation on bone growth in rats. *Ann. N.Y. Acad. Sci.* **114**, Art. 1, 335–338.

Craddock, C. G., Winkelstein, A., Matsuyaki, Y. and Lawrence, J. S. 1967. The immune response to foreign red blood cells and the participation of short lived lymphocytes. *J. Exp. Med.* **125**, 1149–1172.

Crick, F. H. C. 1966. Codon-anticodon pairing: the wobble hypothesis. *J. Mol. Biol.* **19**, 548–555.

Curtis, H. J. 1966. *Biological Mechanisms of Aging.* Charles C. Thomas. Springfield, Ill.

Cutler, S. J., Heise, H. and Eisenberg, H. 1967. Childhood leukemia in Connecticut, 1940–1962. *Blood,* **30**, 1–25.

Czeizel, E., Vaczo, G. and Kertai, P. 1962. Effect of bone-marrow on regeneration of liver of X-irradiated rats. *Nature, Lond.* **196**, 240–241.

Dameshek, W. 1966. Virus induction of autoimmune disease and neoplasia. *Lancet,* **1**, 1268–1269.

—— 1967. Chronic lymphocytic leukaemia – an accumulative disease of immunologically incompetent lymphocytes. *Blood,* **29**, 566–584.

—— and Schwartz, R. S. 1959. Leukemia and auto-immunisation – some possible relationships. *Blood,* **14**, 1151–1158.

Davidson, R. G., Nitowsky, H. N. and Childs, B. 1963. Demonstration of two populations of cells in the human female heterozygous for glucose-6-phosphate dehydrogenase variants. *Proc. Nat. Acad. Sci. U.S.* **50**, 481–485.

Dawson, G. W. P. and Smith-Keary, P. F. 1963. Episomic control of mutation in *Salmonella typhimurium. Heredity,* **18**, 1–20.

Denman, A. M. and Frenkel, E. P. 1967. Studies of the effect of induced immune lymphopenia. I. Enhanced effects of rabbit anti-rat lymphocyte globulin in rats tolerant to rabbit immunoglobulin G. *J. Immunol.* **99**, 498–507.

Deo, M. G., Mathur, M. and Ramalingaswami, V. 1967. Cell regeneration in protein deficiency. *Nature, Lond.* **216**, 499–500.

Dineen, J. K. 1964. Sources of immunological variation. *Nature, Lond.* **202,** 101–102.

Dixon, A. St J. 1968. Familial aspects of gout. In: *University of Edinburgh Pfizer Medical Monographs* 3. *Rheumatic Diseases,* 271–282. J. J. R. Duthie and W. R. M. Alexander (eds.). Edinburgh University Press, Edinburgh.

Dombal, F. T. de 1967a. Private communication.

—— 1967b. The prognostic value of the serum proteins in ulcerative colitis. *Brit. J. Surg.* **54,** 857–859.

——, Watts, J. McK., Watkinson, G. and Goligher, J. C. 1966. Local complications of ulcerative colitis: stricture, pseudopolyposis, and carcinoma of colon and rectum. *Brit. Med. J.* **1,** 1442–1447.

Dubois, E. L. 1966. *Lupus Erythematosis: A Review of the Current Status of Discoid and Systemic Lupus Erythematosus.* Blakiston Division, McGraw-Hill Book Co. Inc., New York.

Early, P. F. 1962. Population studies in Dupuytren's contracture. *J. Bone Jt. Surg.* **44B,** 602–613.

Ederer, F., Myers, M. H. and Mantel, N. 1964. Statistical problems in space and time: do leukemia cases come in clusters? *Biometrics,* **20,** 626–638.

Edwards, F. C. and Truelove, S. C. 1963. The course and prognosis of ulcerative colitis. *Gut,* **4,** 299–315.

Eichwald, E. J. and Silmser, C. R. 1955. Discussion of skin-graft data. *Transpl. Bull.* **2,** 148–149.

Einstein, A. 1949. Autobiographical Notes. In: *Albert Einstein: Philosopher Scientist.* P. A. Schilpp (ed.). Library of Living Philosophers, Evanston, Ill.

Ekstedt, R. D. and Nishimura, E. T. 1964. Runt disease induced in neonatal mice by sterile bacterial vaccines. *J. Exp. Med.* **120,** 795–804.

Elsasser, W. M. 1966. *Atom and Organism. A New Approach to Theoretical Biology.* Princeton University Press, Princeton, New Jersey.

Engel, E. and Forbes, A. P. 1965. Cytogenetic and clinical findings in 48 patients with congenitally defective or absent ovaries. *Medicine,* **44,** 135–164.

Epstein, C. J., Martin, G. M., Schultz, A. L. and Motulsky, A. G. 1966. Werner's syndrome. *Medicine,* **45,** 177–221.

Eriksson, A. W. and Fellman, J. 1967. Twinning in relation to the marital status of the mother. *Acta genet. Basel,* **17,** 385–398.

Fahey, J. L., Finegold, I., Rabson, A. S. and Manaker, R. A. 1966. Immunoglobulin synthesis *in vitro* by established human cell lines. *Science,* **152,** 1259–1261.

Farber, E. M. and Carlsen, R. A. 1966. Psoriasis in childhood. *Calif. Med.* **105,** 415–420.

Feldman, M. and Mekori, T. 1966. Antibody produced by 'cloned' cell populations. *Immunol.* **10,** 149–160.

Fernandez-Herlihy, L. 1959. The articular manifestation of chronic ulcerative colitis. An analysis of 555 cases. *New Engl. J. Med.* **261,** 259–263.

Fialkow, P. J. 1964. Autoimmunity: a predisposing factor to chromosomal aberrations. *Lancet,* **1,** 474–475.

——, Gartler, S. M. and Yoshida, A. 1967. Clonal origin of chronic myelocytic leukemia in man. *Proc. Nat. Acad. Sci. U.S.* **58,** 1468–1471.

Finger, I. and Heller, C. 1964. Cytoplasmic control of gene expression in paramecium. I. Preferential expression of a single allele in heterozygotes. *Genetics,* **49,** 485–498.

Finkel, H. E., Brauer, M. J., Taub, R. N. and Dameshek, W. 1966. Immunologic aberrations in the Di Guglielmo syndrome. *Blood,* **28,** 634–649.

Finn, S. B. 1965. In: *Caries Resistant Teeth.* 41–59. Ciba Foundation Symposium. Churchill, London.

Fisher, J. C. 1958. Multiple-mutation theory of carcinogenesis. *Nature, Lond.* **181,** 651–652.

—— and Hollman, J. H. 1951. A hypothesis of the origin of cancer foci. *Cancer,* **4,** 916–918.

Fitzgerald, M. G. 1967. Clinical aspects of diabetes mellitus. *Abstracts of World Medicine,* **41,** 825–841.

Flaks, A. 1967. Observation of the action of the thymus on the induction of lung tumours by 9,10-Dimethyl-1,2-Benzanthracene (DMBA) in new-born A mice. *Brit. J. Cancer*, **21**, 390–392.

Forbes, A. P. and Engel, E. 1963. The high incidence of diabetes mellitus in 41 patients with gonadal dysgenesis, and their close relatives. *Metabolism*, **12**, 428–439.

Fraumeni, J. F. and Miller, R. W. 1967. Epidemiology of human leukemia: recent observations. *J. Nat. Cancer Inst.* **38**, 593–605.

Freedman, L. R., Blackard, W. G., Sagan, L. A., Ishida, M. and Hamilton, H. B. 1965. The epidemiology of diabetes mellitus in Hiroshima and Nagasaki. *Yale J. Biol. Med.* **37**, 283–299.

Frydman, J. E., Clower, J. W., Fulgham, J. E. and Hester, M. W. 1966. Glaucoma detection in Florida. *J.A.M.A.* **198**, 1237–1240.

Fudenberg, H. N. 1966. Immunologic deficiency, autoimmune disease, and lymphoma: observations, implications and speculations. *Arth. Rheum.* **9**, 464–472.

Fulginiti, V. A., Hathaway, W. E., Pearlman, D. S., Blackburn, W. R., Reiquam, C. W., Githens, J. H., Claman, H. N. and Kempe, C. G. 1966. Dissociation of delayed hypersensitivity and antibody-synthesizing capacities in man. *Lancet*, **2**, 5–8.

Gabr, M., Hashem, N. and Hashem, M. 1960. Progeria, a pathologic study. *J. Pediat.* **57**, 70–77.

Gamow, G. 1967. Does gravity change with time? *Proc. Nat. Acad. Sci. U.S.* **57**, 187–193.

Ganrot, P. O. and Schersten, B. 1967. Serum α_2-macroglobulin concentration and its variation with age and sex. *Clin. Chim. Acta*, **15**, 113–120.

Gartler, S. M., Ziprowski, L., Krakowski, A., Ezra, R., Szeinberg, A. and Adam, A. 1966. Glucose-6-phosphate dehydrogenase mosaicism as a tracer in the study of hereditary multiple trichoepithelioma. *Am. J. Hum. Genet.* **18**, 282–287.

Gaze, R. M. 1967. Growth and differentiation. *Ann. Rev. Physiol.* **29**, 59–86.

Geiduschek, E. P., Tocchini-Valentini, G. P. and Sarnat, M. T. 1964. Asymmetric synthesis of RNA *in vitro*: dependence on DNA continuity and conformation. *Proc. Nat. Acad. Sci. U.S.* **52**, 486–493.

Gill, T. J. 1965. Studies on synthetic polypeptide antigens. XIV Variations in antibody production among rabbits of different inbred strains. *J. Immunol.* **95**, 542–545.

—— and Gershoff, S. N. 1967. The effects of methionine and ethionine on antibody formation in primates. *J. Immunol.* **99**, 883–893.

Good, R. A., Kelly, W. D., Rotstein, J. and Varco, R. L. 1962. Immunological deficiency diseases. *Prog. Allergy*, **6**, 187–319.

Gordon, H. A., Bruckner-Kardoss, E. and Westmann, B. S. 1966. Aging in germ-free mice: life tables and lesions observed at natural death. *J. Gerontol.*, **21**, 380–387.

Gorer, P. A. and Schütze, H. 1938. Genetical studies on immunity in mice. II. Correlation between antibody formation and resistance. *J. Hyg.*, **38**, 647–662.

Green, H. N. 1954. An immunological concept of cancer: a preliminary report. *Brit. Med. J.* **2**, 1374–1380.

—— 1958. Immunological aspects of cancer. In: *Cancer*, **3**, 1–41. R. W. Raven (ed.). Butterworths, London.

Green, I., Litwin, S., Adlersberg, R. and Rubin, I. 1966. Hypogammaglobulinemia with late development of lymphosarcoma. *Arch. Int. Med.*, **118**, 592–602.

—— and Sperber, R. J. 1962. Hypogammaglobulinemia, arthritis, sprue and megaloblastic anemia. *N.Y. State J. Med.* **62**, 1679–1686.

Greenberg, M. 1965. *Studies in Epidemiology*. 184–185. P. B. Rogers (ed.). G. P. Putnam and Sons, New York.

Groth, S. F. de St and Webster, R. G. 1966. Disquisitions on original antigenic sin. *J. Exp. Med.* **124**, 331–345.

Grumbach, M. and Morishima, A. 1964. X chromosome abnormalities in gonadal dysgenesis: DNA replication of structurally abnormal X-chromosome. Relation to thyroid disease. *J. Pediat.* **64**, 1087–1088.

Grüneberg, H. 1966. More about the tabby mouse and about the Lyon hypothesis. *J. Embryol. exp. Morph.* **16**, 569–590.

—— 1967. Sex-linked genes in man and the Lyon hypothesis. *Ann. Hum. Genet. Lond.* **30**, 239–257.

Hale, J. F. and Scowen, E. F. 1967. *Thymic tumours: their Association with Myasthenia Gravis and their Treatment by Radiotherapy.* Lloyd Luke, London.

Hamerton, J. L. 1964. Lyonisation of the X chromosome. *Lancet*, **1**, 1222–1223.

Hanawalt, P. C. and Haynes, R. H. 1967. The repair of DNA. *Scientific American,* **216**, 36–43.

Harris, M. J. and Beveridge, J. 1967. Infectious hepatitis in children. Part 1. General clinical features and progress in 300 patients. *Med. J. Austr.* **2**, 594–596.

Hartman, P. E., Rugis, C. and Stahl, R. C. 1965. Orientation of the histidine operon in the *Salmonella typhimurium* linkage map. *Proc. Nat. Acad. Sci. U.S.* **53**, 1332–1335.

Hayashi, H. and Miura, K-I. 1966. Functional sites in transfer ribonucleic acid. *Nature, Lond.* **209**, 376–378.

Hayes, D. 1967. Mechanism of nucleic acid synthesis. *Ann. Rev. Microbiol.* **21**, 369–382.

Healy, G. M. and Parker, R. C. 1966. Cultivation of mammalian cells in defined media with protein and nonprotein supplements. *J. Cell. Biol.* **30**, 539–553.

Hildemann, W. H. 1957. Scale homotransplantation in goldfish (*Carassius Auratus*). *Ann. N.Y. Acad. Sci.* **64**, 775–791.

Hinuma, Y. and Grace, J. T. 1967. Cloning of immunoglobulin-producing human leukemic and lymphoma cells in long-term cultures. *Proc. Soc. Exp. Biol. Med.* **124**, 107–111.

Hirohata, T., MacMahon, B. and Root, H. F. 1967. The natural history of diabetes. I. Mortality. *Diabetes*, **16**, 875–881.

Hood, L., Gray, W. R. and Dreyer, W. J. 1966. On the evolution of antibody light chains. *J. Mol. Biol.* **22**, 179–182.

Horton, D. L. 1967. The effect of age on hair growth in the CBA mouse: observations on transplanted skin. *J. Gerontol.* **22**, 43–45.

Howard, F. M., Silverstein, M. N. and Mulder, D. W. 1965. The coexistence of myasthenia gravis and pernicious anemia. *Am. J. Med. Sci.* **250**, 518–526.

Hueston, J. T. 1963. *Dupuytren's Contracture.* E. and S. Livingstone Ltd., Edinburgh and London.

Humble, J. G., Jayne, W. H. W. and Pulvertaft, R. J. V. 1956. Biological interaction between lymphocytes and other cells. *Brit. J. Haemat.* **2**, 283–294.

Irvine, W. J., Davies, S. H., Teitelbaum, S., Delamore, I. W. and Wynn Williams, A. 1965. The clinical and pathological significance of gastric parietal cell antibody. *Ann. N.Y. Acad. Sci.* **124**, 657–691.

Isakovié, K., Janković, B. D., Popesković, L. and Milosević, C. 1963. Effect of neonatal thymectomy, bursectomy, and thymo-bursectomy on haemagglutinin production in chickens. *Nature, Lond.* **200**, 273–274.

Jackson, D. 1968. Genes and dental caries. *Proc. Roy. Soc. Med.* **61**, 265–269.

——, Sutcliffe, P. and Burch, P. R. J. 1967. The anatomical site distribution of clinical dental caries in the mandibular incisor teeth of 11- and 12-year-old children. Aetiological implications. *Archs. oral Biol.* **12**, 1343–1353.

Jacob, F. and Monod, J. 1961. Genetic regulatory mechanisms in the synthesis of proteins. *J. Mol. Biol.* **3**, 318–356.

Jansen, C. R., Bond, V. P., Rai, K. R. and Lippincott, S. W. 1964. Abscopal effects of localised irradiation by accelerator beams. *Ann. N.Y. Acad. Sci.* **114**, Art. 1, 302–313.

Jehle, H. L. 1963. Intermolecular forces and biological specificity. *Proc. Nat. Acad. Sci. U.S.* **50**, 516–524.

Jennings, G. H. 1965. Causal influences in haematemesis and melaena. *Gut*, **6**, 1–13.

Jensen, N. K. 1967. Three Danish cases of malignant childhood lymphoma ('Burkitt'). *Acta path. microbiol. Scand.* **70**, 229–235.

Jerne, N. K. 1955. The natural selection theory of antibody formation. *Proc. Nat. Acad. Sci. U.S.* **41**, 849–857.

Joseph, R. R., Zarafonetis, C. J. D. and Durant, J. R. 1966. 'Lymphoma' in chronic granulocytic leukemia. *Am. J. Med. Sci.* **251**, 417–427.

Kabat, E. A. 1967. A comparison of invariant residues in the variable and constant regions of human K, human L, and mouse K Bence-Jones proteins. *Proc. Nat Acad. Sci. U.S.* **58**, 229–233.

Kaliss, N. 1958. Immunological enhancement of tumor homografts in mice. *Cancer Res.* **18**, 992–1003.

—— 1962. The elements of immunologic enhancement: a consideration of mechanisms. *Ann. N.Y. Acad. Sci.* **101**, 64–79.

Kaplan, H. S. and Smithers, D. W. 1959. Auto-immunity in man and homologous disease in mice in relation to the malignant lymphomas. *Lancet*, **2**, 1–4.

Kellum, R. E. and Haserick, J. R. 1964. Systemic lupus erythematosus. *Arch. Int. Med.* **113**, 200–207.

Kerman, R., Segre, D. and Myers, W. L. 1967. Altered response to pneumococcal polysaccharide in offspring of immunologically paralyzed mice. *Science*, **156**, 1514–1516.

Kimball, A. P., Herriot, S. J. and Allinson, P. S. 1967. Studies on immune suppressive drugs. *Proc. Soc. Exp. Biol. Med.* **126**, 181–184.

Klein, E., Klein, G., Nadkarni, J. S., Nadkarni, J. J., Wigzell, A. and Clifford, D. 1967. Surface IgM specificity in cells derived from a Burkitt's lymphoma. *Lancet*, **ii**, 1068–1070.

Kodama, H., Sachin, I. N. and Shabart, E. J. 1967. Rejection of allogeneic skin grafts and alloantibody levels in hyperimmunized mice. *Transplantation*, **5**, 1450–1458.

Kosower, N. S., Vanderhoff, G. A. and London, I. M. 1967. The regeneration of reduced glutathione in normal and glucose-6-phosphate dehydrogenase deficient human red blood cells. *Blood.* **29**, 313–319.

Kubitschek, H. E. 1964. Mutation without segregation. *Proc. Nat. Acad. Sci. U.S.* **52**, 1374–1381.

Lashof, J. C. and Stewart, A. 1965. Oxford survey of childhood cancers. Progress Report III: Leukaemia and Down's syndrome. *Mon. Bull. Min. Hlth.* **24**, 136–143.

Lawrence, J. S., Bremner, J. M. and Bier, F. (1966). Osteo-arthrosis. Prevalence in the population and relationship between symptoms and X-ray changes. *Ann. rheum. Dis.* **25**, 1–24.

Leader, 1967. Outlook in Hodgkin's disease. *Brit. Med. J.* **1**, 328–329.

Lee, J. A. H. 1962. Seasonal variation in the clinical onset of leukaemia in young people. *Brit. Med. J.* **1**, 1737–1738.

Leng, N. and Felsenfeld, G. 1966. The preferential interactions of polylysine and polyarginine with specific base sequences in DNA. *Proc. Nat. Acad. Sci. U.S.* **56**, 1325–1332.

Leong, G. F., Grisham, J. W., Hole, B. V. and Albright, M. L. 1964. Effect of partial hepatectomy on DNA synthesis and mitosis in heterotopic partial autografts of rat liver. *Cancer Res.* **24**, 1496–1501.

Leskowitz, S. 1967. Tolerance. *Ann. Rev. Microbiol.* **21**, 157–180.

Levine, B. B., Ojeda, A. and Benacerraf, B. 1963. Studies on artificial antigens. III. The genetic control of the immune response to hapten-poly-L-lysine conjugates in guinea pigs. *J. Exp. Med.* **118**, 953–957.

Liu, R. K. and Walford, R. L. 1966. Increased growth and life-span with lowered ambient temperature in the annual fish, *Cynolebias adloffi. Nature, Lond.* **212**, 1277–1278.

Loutit, J. F. 1962. Immunological and trophic functions of lymphocytes. *Lancet*, **2**, 1106–1108.

Lyon, M. F. 1961. Genetic action in the X-chromosome of the mouse (*Mus. Musculus L*). *Nature, Lond.* **190**, 372–373.

McCay, C. M. 1952. Chemical aspects of ageing and the effect of diet upon ageing. In: *Problems of Ageing*, 139–202. A. L. Lansing (ed.). Williams and Wilkins Co., Baltimore.

McClintock, B. 1956. Controlling elements and the gene. *Cold Spring Harbour Symp. Quant. Biol.* **21**, 197–206.

McDevitt, H. O. and Sela, M. Genetic control of the antibody response. I. Demonstration of determinant-specific differences in response to synthetic polypeptide antigens in two strains of inbred mice. *J. Exp. Med.* **122**, 517–531.

MacDougall, I. P. M. 1964. The cancer risk in ulcerative colitis. *Lancet*, **2**, 655–658.

McIntire, K. R., Snell, S. and Miller, J. F. A. P. 1964. Pathogenesis of the post-neonatal thymectomy wasting syndrome. *Nature, Lond.* **204**, 151–155.

Mackay, I. A. and Hislop, I. G. 1966. Chronic gastritis and gastric ulcer. *Gut*, **7**, 228–233.

MacMahon, B. 1966. Epidemiology of Hodgkin's disease. *Cancer Res.* **26**, 1189–1200.

—— and Levy, M. A. 1964. Prenatal origin of childhood leukaemia. *New Engl. J. Med.* **270**, 1082–1085.

—— and Newill, V. A. 1962. Birth characteristics of children dying of malignant neoplasms. *J. Nat. Cancer Inst.* **28**, 231–244.

Magnus, H. A. 1952. Gastritis. Chapter 14 in: *Modern Trends in Gastroenterology*, 325–351. F. A. Jones (ed.). Butterworth, London.

Makinodan, T. and Peterson, W. J. 1966. Further studies of the secondary anti-body-forming potential of juvenile, young adult, adult and aged mice. *Develop. Biol.* **14**, 112–129.

Malzberg, B. 1955. Age and sex in relation to mental diseases. *Mental Hygiene*, **39**, 196–224.

Manning, M. D. and Carroll, B. E. 1957. Some epidemiological aspects of leukemia in children. *J. Nat. Cancer Inst.* **19**, 1087–1094.

Margolin, P. 1965. Bipolarity of information transferred from the *Salmonella typhimurium chromosome. Science*, **147**, 1456–1458.

Martinez, C., Kersey, J., Papermaster, B. W. and Good, R. A. 1962. Skin homo-graft survival in thymectomized mice. *Proc. Soc. Exp. Biol. Med.* **109**, 193–196.

Medawar, P. B. 1946. Immunity to homologous grafted skin. II. The relationship between the antigens of blood and skin. *Brit. J. exp. Path.* **27**, 15–24.

Mellon, J. P., Pay, B. Y. and Green, D. M. 1963. Mongolism and thyroid auto-antibodies. *J. ment. Defic. Res.* **7**, 31–37.

Metcalf, D. 1964. Functional interactions between the thymus and other organs. In: *The Thymus*, 53–72. V. Defendi and D. Metcalf (eds.). The Wistar Institute Press, Philadelphia.

Micklem, H. S., Ford, C. E., Evans, E. P. and Gray, J. 1966. Interrelationships of myeloid and lymphoid cells: studies with chromosome-marked cells trans-fused into lethally irradiated mice. *Proc. Roy. Soc. (Lond.)*, **B165**, 78–102.

Miller, D. G. 1967. Immunological deficiency and malignant lymphoma. *Cancer*, **20**, 579–588.

Miller, H., Cendrowski, W. and Schapira, K. 1967. Multiple sclerosis and vaccina-tion. *Brit. Med. J.* **2**, 210–213.

Miller, J. F. A. P. 1962. Effect of neonatal thymectomy on the immunological responsiveness of the mouse. *Proc. Roy. Soc. (Lond.)*, **B156**, 415–428.

—— 1963. Origins of immunological competence. *Brit. Med. Bull.* **19**, 214–218.

Miller, R. W. 1966. Mortality in childhood Hodgkin's disease. *J.A.M.A.* **198**, 1216–1217.

Ministry of Agriculture, 1960 Bulletin: *Disease, Wastage and Husbandry, 1957–1958 in the British Dairy Herd.*

Minowada, J., Klein, G., Clifford, P., Klein, E. and Moore, G. E. 1967. Studies of Burkitt lymphoma cells. *Cancer*, **20**, 1430–1437.

Mitchell, G. F. and Miller, J. F. A. P. 1968. Immunological activity of thymus and thoracic-duct lymphocytes. *Proc. Nat. Acad. Sci. U.S.* **59**, 296–303.

Mitchison, N. A. 1964. Induction of immunological paralysis in two zones of dosage. *Proc. Roy. Soc. (Lond.)*, **B161**, 275–292.

Mittwoch, U. 1967. Sex differentiation in mammals. *Nature, Lond.* **214**, 554–556.

Moolten, F. L. and Bucher, N. L. R. 1967. Regeneration of rat liver: transfer of humoral agent by cross-circulation. *Science*, **158**, 272–274.

Morley, A. A., Baikie, A. G. and Galton, D. A. G. 1967. Cyclic leucocytes as evidence for retention of normal homoeostatic control in chronic granulocytic leukemia. *Lancet*, **2**, 1320–1323.

Mortimer, R., Brustad, T. and Cormack, D. V. 1965. Influence of linear energy transfer and oxygen tension on the effectiveness of ionizing radiations for induction of mutations and lethality in *Saccharomyces cerevisiae*. *Radiation Res.* **26**, 465–482.

Neel, J. V. and Salzano, F. M. 1967. Further studies on the Xavante Indians. X. Some hypotheses – generalizations resulting from these studies. *Am. J. Hum. Genet.* **19**, 554–574.

Neumann, J. von 1955. *The Mathematical Foundations of Quantum Mechanics*. Translated by R. T. Beyer. Princeton University Press, Princeton, New Jersey.

Neumayer, E., Perger, F., Schinko, H. and Tschabitscher, H. 1956. Das serumeiweissbild bei der multiplen sklerose. *Wien. Z. NervHeilk.* **13**, 46–64.

Neyman, J. 1967. R. A. Fisher (1890–1962): an appreciation. *Science*, **156**, 1456–1460.

Nielsen, J. 1966a. Diabetes mellitus in parents of patients with Klinefelter's syndrome. *Lancet*, **1**, 1376.

—— 1966b.Twins in sibships with Klinefelter's syndrome. *J. Med. Genet.* **3**, 114–116.

Nirenberg, M., Leder, P., Bernfield, M., Brimacombe, R., Trupin, J., Rottman, F. and O'Neal, C. 1965. RNA codewords and protein synthesis. VII. On the general nature of the RNA code. *Proc. Nat. Acad. Sci. U.S.* **53**, 1161–1168.

Nora, J. J., Gilliland, J. C., Sommerville, R. J. and McNamara, D. G. 1967. Congenital heart disease in twins. *New Engl. J. Med.* **277**, 568–571.

Nossal, G. J. V. 1967. Mechanisms of antibody production. *Ann. Rev. Medicine*, **18**, 81–96.

——, Szenberg, A., Ada, G. L. and Austin, C. M. 1964. Single cell studies on 19S antibody production. *J. Exp. Med.* **119**, 485–502.

Novick, A. and Szilard, L. 1950. Experiments with the chemostat on spontaneous mutations of bacteria. *Proc. Nat. Acad. Sci. U.S.* **36**, 708–719.

Oleinick, A. 1967. Leukemia or lymphoma occurring subsequent to an autoimmune disease. *Blood*, **29**, 144–153.

O'Reilly, S. 1967. Problems in Wilson's disease. *Neurology*, **17**, 137–146.

Osgood, E. E. 1957. A unifying concept of the etiology of the leukemias, lymphomas, and cancer. *J. Nat. Cancer Inst.* **18**, 155–166.

—— 1964. The etiology of leukemias, lymphomas, and cancers. *Geriatrics*, **19**, 208–221.

Panse, F. 1942. *Die Erbchorea*. George Thieme Verlag, Leipzig.

Paronetto, F., Horowitz, R. E., Sicular, A., Burrows, L., Kark, A. E. and Popper, A. 1965. Immunologic observations on homografts. I. The canine liver. *Transplantation*, **3**, 303–317.

Parrott, D. M. V. and East, J. 1962. Role of the thymus in neonatal life. *Nature, Lond.* **195**, 347–348.

Peacock, E. E. and Biggars, W. P. 1962. Changes in plasma proteins of mice during rejection of skin homografts and heterografts. *Proc. Soc. Exp. Biol. Med.* **111**, 131–133.

Pelc, S. R. 1965. Correlation between coding-triplets and amino-acids. *Nature, Lond.* **207**, 597–599.

Peterson, R. D. A., Cooper, M. D. and Good, R. A. 1965. The pathogenesis of immunologic deficiency diseases. *Am. J. Med.* **38**, 579–604.

—— —— —— 1967. Disorders of the thymus and other lymphoid tissues. In: *Progress in Medical Genetics*. 1–31. A. G. Bear and A. G. Steinberg (eds.). Grune and Stratton Inc., New York.

Pike, M. C., Williams, E. H. and Wright, B. 1967. Burkitt's tumour in the West Nile district of Uganda 1961–6. *Brit. Med. J.* **2**, 395–399.

Pinchuk, P. and Maurer, P. H. 1965. Antigenicity of polypeptides (poly alpha amino acids). XVI. Genetic control of immunogenicity of synthetic polypeptides in mice. *J. Exp. Med.* **122**, 673–679.

Platt, Lord. 1967. Medical science: master or servant? *Brit. Med. J.* **iii**, 439–444.

Porter, K. A., Thomson, W. B., Owen, K., Kenyon, J. R., Mowbray, J. F. and Peart, W. S. 1963. Obliterative vascular changes in four human kidney homotransplants. *Brit. Med. J.* **2**, 639–645.

Portier, P. and Richet, C. 1902. De l'action anaphylactique de certains renins. *C.R. Soc. Biol.* **54**, 170–172.

Ptashne, M. 1967. Specific binding of the λ phage repressor to λ DNA. *Nature, Lond.* **214**, 232–234.

Pulvertaft, C. N. 1965. Private communication.

Putnam, F. W., Shinoda, T., Titani, K. and Wikler, M. 1967. Immunoglobulin structure: variation in amino acid sequence and length of human lambda light chains. *Science,* **157**, 1050–1053.

Registrar General, 1958. *Statistical Review of England and Wales for the Year 1956.* Part III. Commentary. H.M.S.O., London.

—— 1963. *Statistical Review of England and Wales for the Year 1961.* Part I. Tables. Medical. H.M.S.O., London.

Reimann, H. A. 1962. Hereditary periodic edema. The interrelation of familial periodic disorders. *Am. J. Med. Sci.* **243**, 727–739.

Richards, W., Siegel, S. C., Strauss, J. and Leigh, M. D. 1967. Status asthmaticus in children. *J.A.M.A.* **201**, 75–81.

Ripps, C. S. and Hirschhorn, K. 1967. The production of immunoglobulins by human peripheral blood lymphocytes *in vitro. Clin. exp. Immunol.* **2**, 377–398.

Ritzmann, S. E., Stoufflet, E. J., Houston, E. W. and Levin, W. C. 1966. Coexistent chronic myelocytic leukemia, monoclonal gammopathy and multiple chromosomal abnormalities. *Am. J. Med.* **41**, 981–989.

Rose, J. E. M. St and Cinader, B. 1967. The effect of tolerance on the specificity of the antibody response and on immunogenicity. Antibody response to conformationally and chemically altered antigens. *J. Exp. Med.* **125**, 1031–1055.

Rose, N. R. and Witebsky, E. 1956. Studies on organ specificity. V. Changes in the thyroid glands of rabbits following active immunization with rabbit thyroid extracts. *J. Immunol.* **76**, 417–427.

Rosenberg, S. A. and Kaplan, H. S. 1966. Evidence for an orderly progression in the spread of Hodgkin's disease. *Cancer Res.* **26**, 1225–1231.

Rous, P. 1967. The challenge to man of the neoplastic cell. *Science,* **157**, 24–28.

Rowell, N. R. and Beck, J. S. 1967. Antinuclear factors. *Brit. Med. J.* **3**, 307.

Rubin, P. 1966. Controversial issues in the treatment of Hodgkins's disease. *Progress in Hematology,* **5**, 180–203.

Russell, W. L. 1964. In: *Genetics Today.* Proc. XI International Congress on Genetics The Hague, The Netherlands. Pergamon Press.

—— 1965. Studies in mammalian radiation genetics. *Nucleonics,* **23**, 53–56 and 62.

Sampson, D. and Archer, G. T. 1967. Release of histamine from human basophils. *Blood,* **29**, 722–736.

Sanderson, K. E. 1965. Information transfer in *Salmonella typhimurium Proc. Nat. Acad. Sci. U.S.* **53**, 1335–1340.

Schaller, J., Davis, D. S. and Wedgwood, R. J. 1966. Failure of development of the thymus, lymphopenia and hypogammaglobulinemia. *Am. J. Med.* **41**, 462–472.

Scheibel, I. F. 1943. Hereditary differences in capacity of guinea pigs for production of diphtheria antitoxin. *Acta path. microbiol., Scand.* **20**, 464–484.

Schneer, J. H. 1967. Pseudomosaicism and G-6-PD deficiency. *Lancet,* **ii**, 466–467.

Seldam, R. E. J., Cooke, R. and Atkinson, L. 1966. Childhood lymphoma in the territories of Papua and New Guinea. *Cancer,* **19**, 437–446.

Shelley, W. B. and Arthur, R. P. 1958. Biochemical and physiological clues to the nature of psoriasis. *Arch. Derm.* **78**, 14–29.

Shelley, W. B. and Parnes, H. M. 1965. The absolute basophil count. *J.A.M.A.* **192**, 368–370.

Sherman, J. D. and Dameshek, W. 1963. 'Wasting disease' following thymectomy in the hamster. *Nature, Lond.* **197**, 469–471.

Shipley, P. W., Wray, J. A., Hechter, H. H., Arellano, M. G. and Borhani, N. O. 1967. Frequency of twinning in California. *Am. J. Epidem.* **85**, 147–156.

Sloan, W. P., Bargen, J. A. and Gage, R. O. 1950. Life histories of patients with chronic ulcerative colitis: a review of 2000 cases. *Gastroenterology*, **16**, 25–38.

Smithers, D. W. 1967. Hodgkin's disease. *Brit. Med. J.* **2**, 263–268.

Smithies, O. 1967. Antibody variability. *Science*, **157**, 267–273.

Sobey, W. R. 1954. The inheritance of antibody response to tobacco mosaic virus in rabbits. *Austr. J. Biol. Sci.* **7**, 111–117.

——, Magrath, J. M. and Reisner, A. H. 1966. Genetically controlled immunological unresponsiveness. *Immunol.* **11**, 511–513.

Sohar, E., Gafni, J. Pras, M. and Heller, H. 1967. Familial Mediterranean fever. *Am. J. Med.* **43**, 227–253.

Song, J. H. and Sobey, W. R. 1954. The genetic control of response to antigenic stimuli. *J. Immunol.* **72**, 52–65.

Sparkes, R. S. and Motulsky, A. G. 1963. Hashimoto's disease in Turner's syndrome with isochromosome X. *Lancet*, **1**, 947.

Spencer, R. P. and Coulombe, M. J. 1966. Quantitation of hepatic growth and regeneration. *Growth*, **30**, 277–284.

Spiegelman, M. and Marks, H. H. 1946. Age and sex variations in prevalence and onset of diabetes mellitus. *Am. J. Pub. Hlth* **36**, 26–33.

Stark, C. R. and Mantel, N. 1966. Effects of maternal age and birth order on the risk of mongolism and leukemia. *J. Nat. Cancer Inst.* **37**, 687–698.

Stewart, A. 1967. Private communication.

—— Webb, J. and Hewitt, D. 1958. A survey of childhood malignancies. *Brit. Med. J.* **1**, 1495–1508.

Stromberg, L. R., Woodward, K. T., Maghin, D. T. and Donati, R. M. 1967. Altered wound healing in X-irradiated rats: the effect of bone marrow shielding. *Experientia*, **23**, 1064–1065.

Swann, M. M. 1957. The control of cell division: a review. I. General mechanisms. *Cancer Res.* **17**, 727–757.

—— 1958. The control of cell division: a review. II. Special mechanisms. *Cancer Res.* **18**, 1118–1160.

Szenberg, A. and Warner, N. L. 1962. Dissociation of immunological responsiveness in fowls with a hormonally arrested development of lymphoid tissues. *Nature, Lond* **194**, 146–147.

Taverner, D. 1965. Private communication.

——, Fearnley, M. E., Kemble, F., Miles, D. W. and Peiris, O. A. 1966. Prevention of denervation in Bell's palsy. *Brit. Med. J.* **1**, 391–393.

——, Kemble, F. and Cohen, S. B. 1967. Prognosis and treatment of idiopathic facial (Bell's) palsy. *Brit. Med. J.* **4**, 581–582.

Taylor, K., Hradecna, Z. and Szybalski, W. 1967. Asymmetric distribution of the transcribing regions on the complementary strands of coliphage λ DNA. *Proc. Nat. Acad. Sci.* **57**, 1618–1625.

Taylor, P. E., Tejada, C. and Sáuchez, M. 1967. The effect of malnutrition on the inflammatory response. *J. Exp. Med.* **126**, 539–555.

Thompson, D.' A. W. 1952. (Reprinted) *Growth and Form*— Cambridge University Press, London.

Thompson, H. 1965. Abnormalities of the autosomal chromosome associated with human disease: selected topics and catalogue. *Am. J. Med. Sci.* **250**, 718–735.

Till, M. M., Hardisty, R. M., Pike, M. C. and Doll, R. 1967. Childhood leukaemia in Greater London: a search for evidence of clustering. *Brit. Med. J.* **3**, 755–758.

Trentin, J., Wolf, N., Cheng, V., Fahlberg, W., Weiss, D. and Bonhag, R. 1967. Antibody production by mice repopulated with limited numbers of clones of lymphoid cell precursors. *J. Immunol.* **98**, 1326–1337.

Troup, G. M. and Walford, R. L. 1967. Transplantation disease, renal lysozyme, and aging. *Transplantation*, **5**, 43–50.

Twomey, J. J., Levin, W. C., Melnick, M. B., Trobaugh, F. E. and Allgood, J. W. 1967. Laboratory studies on a family with a father and son affected by acute leukemia. *Blood* **29**, 920–930.

Tyan, M. L. and Cole, L. J. 1964. Sources of potential immunologically reactive cells in certain foetal and adult tissues. *Transplantation*, **2**, 241–245.

—— 1967. An impairment of antibody production in adoptively restored, lethally irradiated thymectomized mice. *Clin. exp. Immunol.* **2**, 121–131.

Tyler, A. 1947. An auto-antibody concept of cell structure, growth and differentiation. *Sixth Growth Symposium*, 7–19. The Heffernan Press, Worcester, Mass.

Ultmann, J. E., Cunningham, J. K. and Gellhorn, A. 1966. The clinical picture of Hodgkin's disease. *Cancer Res.* **26**, 1047–1060.

Upton, A. C., Conte, F. P., Hurst, G. S. and Mells, W. A. 1956. The relative biological effectiveness of neutrons, X-rays and gamma-rays for acute lethality in mice. *Radiation Res.* **4**, 117–131.

Ustvedt, H. J. 1958. Ulcerative colitis in Norway. In: *Recent Studies in Epidemiology*, J. Pemberton and H. Willard (eds.). Blackwell Scientific Publications, Oxford.

Vazquez, J. J. and Makinodan, T. 1966. Cytokinetic events following antigenic stimulation. *Fed. Proc.* **25**, 1727–1733.

Virolainen, N. 1964. Mitotic response in liver autograt after partial hepatectomy in the rat. *Exp. Cell Res.* **33**, 388–391.

Wachtel, L. W. and Cole, L. J. 1965. Abscopal effects of whole-body X-irradiation on compensatory hypertrophy of the rat kidney. *Radiation Res.* **25**, 1272–1274.

Walford, R. L. 1962. Auto-immunity and aging. *J. Gerontol.* **17**, 281–285.

—— 1967. The role of autoimmune phenomena in the ageing process. In: *Aspects of the Biology of Ageing*, 351–373. H. W. Woolhouse (ed.). *Symp. Soc. Exp. Biol.*, No. 21, Cambridge University Press, London.

Way, S. 1954. Aetiology of cancer of body of the uterus. *J. Obstet. Gynaec. Brit. Emp.* **61**, 46–48.

Weber, W. T. 1966. Difference between medullary and cortical thymic lymphocytes of the pig in their response to phytohemagglutinin. *J. Cell. Physiol.* **68**, 117–125.

Weigert, M. C. and Garen, A. 1965. Base composition of nonsense codons in *E. coli*. Evidence from amino acid substitutions at a tryptophan site in alkaline phosphatase. *Nature, Lond.* **206**, 992–994.

Weinstein, I. B. 1963. Comparative studies on the genetic code. *Cold Spring Harbour Symp. Quant. Biol.* **28**, 579–580.

Weiss, P. A. 1947. The problem of specificity in growth and development. *Yale J. Biol. Med.* **19**, 235–278.

—— 1950. Perspectives in the field of morphogenesis. *Q. Rev. Biol.* **25**, 177–198.

—— 1955. Specificity in growth control. In: *Biological Specificity and Growth*, 195–206. E. G. Butler (ed.). Princeton University Press, Princeton, New Jersey.

—— 1962. Cells and their environment including other cells. Chapter 1 in: *Biological Interactions in Normal and Neoplastic Growth*, 3–20. Little Brown and Co. (Inc.), New York.

—— and Kavanau, J. L. 1957. A model of growth and growth control in mathematical terms. *J. Gen. Physiol.* **41**, 1–47.

West, C. D., Fowler, R. and Nathan, P. 1960. The relationship of serum globulin to transplant rejection in the dog studied by paper and immunoelectrophoretic techniques. *Ann. N.Y. Acad. Sci.* **87**, 522–537.

Westlund, K. 1966. Incidence of diabetes mellitus in Oslo, Norway 1925 to 1954. *Brit. J. Prev. Soc. Med.* **20**, 105–116.

Whitehouse, H. L. K. 1967. Crossover model of antibody variability. *Nature, Lond.* **215**, 371–374.

Wigley, R. G. and Maclaurin, B. P. 1962. A study of ulcerative colitis in New Zealand, showing a low incidence in Maoris. *Brit. Med. J.* **ii**, 228–231.

Wilson, D. B. 1967. Lymphocytes as mediators of cellular immunity: destruction of homologous target cells in culture. *Transplantation*, **5**, 986–988.

Witebsky, E. and Rose, N. R. 1956. Studies on organ specificity. IV. Production of rabbit thyroid antibodies in the rabbit. *J. Immunol.* **76**, 408–416.

Witte, J. J. and Karchmer, A. W. 1968. Surveillance of mumps in the United States as background for use of vaccine. *Public Health Reports*, **83**, 95–100.

Woese, C. R. 1965. Order in the genetic code. *Proc. Nat. Acad. Sci. U.S.* **54**, 71–75.

——, Dugre, D. H., Saxinger, W. C. and Dugre, S. A. 1966. The molecular basis for the genetic code. *Proc. Nat. Acad. Sci. U.S.* **55**, 966–974.

Yarus, M. and Berg, P. 1967. Recognition of tRNA by aminoacyl tRNA synthetases. *J. Mol. Biol.* **28**, 479–490.

Yoffey, J. M. 1966. *Bone Marrow Reactions*. Edward Arnold (Publishers) Ltd., London.

INDEX